M000219711

BREAKTHROUGH FOR DYSLEXIA AND LEARNING DISABILITIES

BREAKTHROUGH FOR DYSLEXIA AND LEARNING DISABILITIES

CARL A. FERRERI, D.C., PH.C.
AND
RICHARD B. WAINWRIGHT, D.C., PH.C.

Illustrated by Ron Thomson

Exposition Press of Florida, Inc.
Pompano Beach, Florida

FIRST EDITION

Library of Congress Catalog Card Number: 84-090414

ISBN 0-682-40186-2

Printed in the United States of America

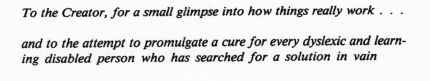

To the Creator, for a small glimpse into how things really work . . .

and to the attempt to promulgate a cure for every dyslexic and learning disabled person who has searched for a solution in vain

Contents

Foreword

When Dr. Wainwright asked me to write a foreword for this historic book, I was quite flattered. As I began to organize my thoughts, I came to realize the deeper meaning and significance to the vast millions of individuals who suffer from the afflictions of learning disabilities and dyslexia. The patients who already have sought help from Drs. Ferreri and Wainwright have a shared past and a happier future now.

In order to comprehend the milestone that these patients have attained, the reader must understand just what these afflictions can do to a person's life.

For the adult patient who is now in his thirties, his problem was barely understood by the educational world when he was of school age. Whether he was a sufferer of dyslexia or a milder form of learning disablement, the educational establishment, in most cases, chose to ignore the problem or, in many instances, would blame the child, the parent, or both for his shortcomings. If the parents were aggressive and not accepting of the school's "washing of the hands," they would seek out physicians for aid and advice, only to be informed that there were no organic deficits or other apparent causes for the child's inability to learn. Some children, however, did benefit from checkups and evaluations of previously undetected medical problems that were discovered, diagnosed, and corrected. They were the lucky few. The majority were not so fortunate and were left to scramble as best they could. Medicine offered two possibilities to explain why a youngster was learning disabled. He was suffering from some form of visual dysfunction or perhaps an auditory deficit.

Treatments that were rendered demonstrated improvement and

gave hope to both the patient and his family. Unfortunately, these improvements turned out to be of short duration and the deficits remained.

In school, their nightmare continued unabated. Their frustration began early in grammar school. Reading, writing, and math—which make up our all-important foundation in this technological age— were the first betrayers to our sufferers. Letters never seemed to remain constant; they changed form and appeared differently. To the chagrin of the youngster, words got scrambled or actually disappeared, or parts were missing or were juxtaposed. It was madness to ask a child to develop a successful test performance and build his educational foundation over a pool of quicksand. There just was no stability to work with.

When the child wrote, the letters, words, and sentences became nothing more than a jumbled mess that frequently seemed to flow all over the paper. The handwriting was erratic at best. The written expression was illiterate at worst. In math, the child fared no better. Numbers seemed to have a mind of their own. They would move at random. Lines or signs began to merge or run away on the paper. At no time could a student or teacher expect constancy in a lesson. The norm for this type of student was failure—failure on tests, quizzes, classwork, and homework—failure in everything.

Failures in all areas of schoolwork, however, didn't always occur for all students. Sometimes a child might succeed in sports, others in work that demanded less academic preparation, and a minimal number of students did succeed in getting better than passing grades. Those lucky few were of more than average intelligence and had the ability to compensate for their deficits. Amazingly, a student might even become a college graduate. Mostly, this was accomplished under the most strenuous and painfully arduous exertions.

Has special education made a difference for today's learning disabled or dyslexic student? The answer is both yes and no. Yes, special education has helped immensely. Today's young student is tested and quickly evaluated by many professionals as being learning disabled or dyslexic. At that point, a teacher, trained in special education, sets up a program aimed at improving the areas that this type of child functions in best. For example, a child who has trouble with visual perception would receive all classwork in an auditory mode and through tactile sensation. His education program has been modified to take advantage of his areas of best performance, while he also is taught how to come to grips with his learning deficits. In no way has this child become nondyslexic or nonlearning disabled.

Through the active intervention of the authors' potentiation of the documented case histories in this book, each patient experienced a lessening of his or her disability. Their treatment aims at the very heart of the cause of the learning disabled. Potentiation has opened the door for these patients, enabling them to lead a normal life for the first time. This brings to mind a patient who, upon leaving the office after receiving his first treatment, exclaimed, "So that's what a tree looks like." Never before had he seen a three-dimensional tree. For him it had been a one-dimensional world.

Indeed with pride, I heartily recommend to anyone suffering or knowing of anyone suffering from a learning disability or dyslexia that there is now real help for you, and to read on.

Marc M. Nagelberg, B.A., Ms.Ed., C.A.S.
Past Director, Adult Education Dept.
Educational Specialist in Emotionally,
Mentally, and Learning Disabled

Preface

1. Do you confuse the addition and multiplication signs or the subtraction and division signs?
2. Do you tend to run into things even though you try to avoid them?
3. Do you confuse your right and left?
4. Do you occasionally write or print backward or reverse your letters?
5. Do you read or talk with any degree of hesitation?
6. Is your walk unsmooth or disorganized?
7. Do you have short-span memory retention?
8. Do directional signs confuse you?
9. Do you have to ask people to repeat conversations because you're not sure what they said?
10. Do you get lost when trying to follow directions to a location?
11. Do you lose or skip lines while reading?
12. Do you lose the sense of what you are reading?

If you must answer any of the above questions with a "yes" for either yourself or your child, it is very possible that you are among the twenty percent of the population who are said to have some degree of learning disability.[2]*

*Footnote number refers to bibliographical entry.

Introduction

The most recent addition to the practice of chiropractic is that of applied kinesiology. Kinesiology as a subject has been around for a long time, but only as a study of body motion. It took Dr. George Goodheart to correlate the myriad bits of information available and put them into a usable system, which is now known as applied kinesiology. It is a system in which the degree of muscle tone or strength is used to indicate the integrity of the muscle, the part or a particular circuit or function in the body. Applied kinesiology wears many hats. It indicates to the doctor or examiner that a certain function, part, or movement is at fault. It also indicates the treatment necessary to make the correction and, finally, demonstrates if the correction was or wasn't accomplished.

The basic treatment procedures have evolved from many sources and many disciplines but have been brought together under one roof by Goodheart.[1]

With the understanding that kinesiology is the study of motion, we can expand our thinking and examine some basic terminology.

kinetics:	study of motion
kinesiology:	study of body motion
applied kinesiology:	study of body motion and what it means
hypokinesis:	diminished body movement—less than that which is considered to be normal, such as lethargy
hyperkinesis:	increased body movement—more than that which is considered to be normal, such as hyperactivity

It is hoped that the first of these words, kinetics, will be very much a part of us all of our lives. Without motion of the many parts of the body, life would terminate rather soon, so it behooves us to ensure motion at all cost.

The fourth and fifth words, hypokinesis and hyperkinesis, deal with motion also but not of a normal amount. The infant, child, or adult who has hypo problems will show practically no emotion, no enthusiasm, and will be shortchanged in energy. They will lag behind in group activity, will be whiners, and will drag through mealtime until the dessert course arrives.

The hyper person, comparatively, is highly emotional and is on the lookout continually for active things, as a matter of fact, risky things to do. The expressed energy is boundless. The hyper person will bubble up to the top and try to take over the leadership in groups; they communicate with shouts and screams. In relating a story the hyper person will describe events in superlatives, often resorting to out-and-out lies to embellish a situation. When a parent speaks of her child as "off the wall," she is speaking of a child with hyperkinesis.

Applied kinesiology is used to test for and treat many conditions, a large number of which have defeated health providers until recently. The procedure is spreading rapidly and, we are glad to report, is now being utilized by members of other healing arts, i.e., dentists, ophthalmologists, psychiatists, and holistic doctors of various disciplines. It is exciting to see historically competitive schools of thought coming together and meeting on common ground. Only good can come of this, and the patient is the beneficiary.

One of the most bothersome conditions plaguing children, and adults as well, is the catchall conglomeration known as "learning disabilities." The purpose of this book is to address this situation from an analytical, as well as the therapeutic, point of view.

Acknowledgments

Some time ago someone said, "No man is an island." I was fortunate to come into contact with many teachers, writers, discoverers, and innovators along the way who found functions in the body not known previously. They postulated new ideas and concepts and were not satisfied with the accepted knowledge of how the body works. They questioned, researched, experimented, and, in almost all cases, spent their own monies and time to find what needed to be known. They never were satisfied; nothing ever was good enough. More had to be known. The establishment was not giving the answers, particularly for the average person, who had less than exotic conditions or health problems.

I have to thank the tireless, unselfish efforts of men like Dr. Major Bertram DeJarnette for his more than fifty years of research and teaching, resulting in the marvelous sacro-occipital and cranial techniques, and Dr. George Goodheart, formerly a disciple of the "Major," for his discovery and development, over the last twenty years, of what is known as applied kinesiology. These two men have advanced the knowledge of how the body really works by at least 2,000 years. They certainly are deserving of the Nobel Prize for their contributions to the human race.

Others who deserve praise for their efforts are Dr. John Thie of California, who made kinesiology logical for me; Dr. David Denton of California, who made sure I understood the cranial and other functions, along with Dr. David Walther in their teaching efforts at the Parker Research and other seminars; Dr. Melvin Reese of Sedan, Kansas, and Dr. Stanley Wieczorek of Fancher, New York, for their encouragement, innovativeness, and fantastic knowledge;

Dr. Herbert Anderson of Medford, Massachusetts, for his dedication and willingness to share his vast knowledge and experience; Drs. Jose Rodriguez, Salvatore Cordaro, and Lawrence De Mann for their early teaching efforts; and, finally, all the men and women who unselfishly dedicated their time at the Parker and Omaha seminars through the years.

Special thanks are due to my first technique instructor, Dr. Martin I. Phillips (fifty years ahead of his time and unaware of it), who was responsible for my eye muscle technique, and Dr. Richard B. Wainwright, who was instrumental in my becoming a chiropractor in the first place. With much personal sacrifice, he is coauthoring this book with me.

Dr. Carl A. Ferreri

1

The Learning Disabled

It has been known by many researchers for more than eighty-five years that "learning disability" is a valid, classified condition.[3] Up until 1896, children had their ears boxed or were otherwise punished when they carried out directions or instructions in ways other than what was wanted. Pity the poor child whose next meal depended on whether he followed orders as given or with his own improper or misunderstood interpretation. Grieve for the lad who had the overpowering urge to follow the mast, only to discover that his inability to interpret orders as given by his captain resulted in floggings, even to the point of death. He was at sea all right, but without the slightest chance of improvement of his lot.

Can the man who strongly desires to work with horses but can't appreciate distance, colors, depth, or speed expect anything more than a stableman's job?

One poor soul comes to mind from out of the past—an Irish girl who had been sponsored by a family near by was trying valiantly to do all the right things as a servant. This was important because failure could result in being returned home to her impoverished hovel near the mines. She probably would have managed like many other immigrants if she had had a patient employer and if she did not have the misfortune of being what we now know to be dyslexic. By the time the poor girl tried to cope with bettering her English, suffering the frustration of mixing up instructions, twisting directions, and reading what wasn't there, and then adding to that the humiliation

1

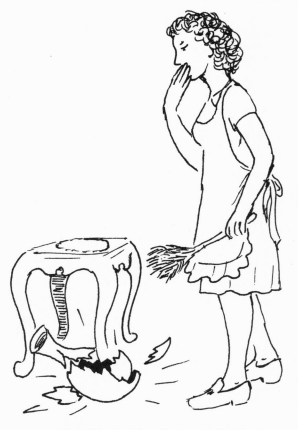

A small accident with a deep-seated reason

of being bawled out by the housewife who certainly should have known better, one would think the girl would have been far happier tending her small garden, having not ever left Ireland in the first place. She might not have accomplished very much else, but she would have been calm and safe.

Until recently, this type of behavior was considered obstinate, disobedient, noncaring, lazy, stupid, mentally retarded, as well as

other unfortunate adjectives. We now know that these are manifestations of a category of conditions referred to as learning disabilities.
These are many-faceted conditions, neurologically involving more
than the obvious learning or performing problems. Probably the most
complicated of these is that of dyslexia. This condition has perplexed
investigators for almost a century. Dyslexia would not stand still long
enough for anyone to categorize. It was almost never the same in
the particular patient being examined. The only thing that seemed
to be consistent was that all dyslexics invert or see and/or write things
backward at least some of the time. They have an inability to follow
printed or written lines from one to the other. They are confused
as to the proper position on a page. They seem to confuse instructions and never remember right from left. Some note that they are
discoordinated in gait or hand/eye coordination. It has been noted
that there seems to be a disequilibrium, *not* vertigo but a gentle
"rocking of the boat." Other investigators have pointed out an apparent problem in comprehending the spoken word. Many children
and adults, therefore, speak with difficulty as if they were slightly
deaf. Vowels are flat, run together, or, in some cases, almost
eliminated. Understanding what is being said by a dyslexic is, at
times, very difficult. Just as the *condition* of dyslexia is difficult to
diagnose, so the dyslexic himself is hard to pin down as to what
his problem really is. The manifestations are not consistent.
Sometimes he writes "was," sometimes "saw," sometimes "asw."
They are almost never the same.

Some dyslexics can perform certain very intricate hand/eye functions
and seem to be able to put anything together or take it apart. Others
become proficient in some sports activity or become excellent dancers.
Many investigators tend to segment the definitions and not consider all
the factors as part of the total problem with many manifestations.

In the main, people with dyslexia cannot read, cannot read well,
or find it very difficult, if not impossible, to read aloud. Usually
they cannot compose a proper letter or paragraph. Most have poor
comprehension of what they attempt to read. They often find
mathematics effortful if not impossible (particularly with number
reversals). They will avoid any type of sports where they have to
hit, catch, or kick a ball. They usually are loners or have very few

friends who will be inferior intellectually or will be those not requiring interaction on anything but a superficial basis. Most are clumsy, bump into and/or drop things. They generally have poor directional sense, get lost easily, or forget why they were heading in a particular direction. They have poor comprehension, and many are slow in speech because they have to try very hard to compose an intelligent sentence. They tend to reverse instructions as they do letters, words, and numbers. They appear to be moody, preoccupied, obstinate, sometimes stupid or even mentally deficient, when actually they are confused, frustrated, embarrassed, desperate, and afraid.

Fortunately, there are ways of overcoming these sad situations. Applied kinesiology has stepped in to save the day and aid the problem. Recent research by chiropractic kinesiologists has brought to light an astoundingly rapid solution to the abysmal load the learning disabled have had to bear.

Through rather simple structural and neurological analyses, the root of the problem is determined and the correction is made virtually then and there in an appreciable number of cases. The examination embraces many aspects of investigation that have been considered in past years by various learning institutions, but that is where the similarity ends.

Applied kinesiology is then put into gear. Cloacal reflex points are checked, cranial faults are explored, cervical alignment is checked, and the temporal-mandibular joints are examined. Gait mechanisms are considered and right or left dominance is checked. Nothing is left out in determining the basic reasons for the disability, and the procedure is repeated until the patient is asymptomatic. The authors have found that, on the average, this occurs by the third to the eighth treatment.[24]

Subtle degrees of academic disability may not be spotted early on, and the child might be passed along to his next learning chore not having completed development in his last one. Before long there is a piling up of deficiencies that may be impossible to catch up with. In later years, many adults still saddled with the problem have acclimated themselves, have learned many tricks in order to mask their affliction, and in too many instances will out and out refuse to recognize that a problem exists at all. This certainly is not something to be ashamed of but surely is something to be dealt with, the sooner the better.

Obviously the younger the child the easier the case. Once the child has been forced through several grades, he or she will have a lot of catching up to do in the three Rs. Letters won't behave; numbers won't stand still. One moment a sign says "do" or "27" or "can," the next moment the same sign says "don't" or "72" or "can't." The learning disabled person is never quite sure which is real, so he or she has worked out subterfuges to rationalize an educated (sic) guess. All goes well until a crisis decision has to be made; here is where trouble, injury, or embarrassment comes about. Either the person is unable to carry out an order, has a traumatic experience, or appears to be lacking in the qualities his or her peers thought he or she possessed.

It has been found that the chance of the parent with a disability, producing a child with the same condition is very high. The malady seems to follow through a familial line quite readily. Ann Bradford Mathias, wife of Sen. Charles Mathias of Maryland, is a direct descendant of William Bradford, governor of the Plymouth Colony in the 1600s. One of her cousins, Dr. Edwin Cole, founder of the language training program at Massachusetts General Hospital, traced Ann's lineage and found learning disability had dogged the family for about 300 years.

Mrs. Mathias is now concerned about her younger son, Rob, who is showing signs of a similar disorder.[4] It would be the height of cruelty for the afflicted parent to disregard watching the child very carefully because of some misguided notion that he had something to hide. The parent with the problem should pay special attention to his offspring; they run a higher risk than other children. It would be nothing short of tragedy to waste a mind through carelessness when the solution is so near to all of us.

When colleges form dyslexia clubs in an attempt to deal with the students' shortcomings, it easily can be seen that a genuine problem exists, but forewarned is forearmed. The various learning disabilities, and dyslexia is one of the most serious, should be ferreted out and properly treated the first moment they appear. The child should not have to wait until he is forced to seek a solution on his own. The chiropractic profession has developed an answer to an old problem, and the fact should be taken advantage of at the earliest possible opportunity.

It is, of course, a wonderful thing that has been done by the many associations, groups, concerned researchers, and dedicated teachers in spending unending time with the learning disabled. They work with them practically from the cradle right on through adulthood. They have drilled, coached, wheedled, begged, and demanded; the hapless students have given all they had to give. Unfortunately, it has not been enough; some ingredient was lacking. That is all changing now. Unremitting effort has gone into research and exciting gains have been accomplished. The available statistics in the authors' files are encouraging, especially when one finds that virtually all of the cases posted have shown excellent improvement, and most have resulted in complete clearance of all symptoms.

It must be understood that the brain damaged and mentally retarded are not included in this work.

The following definition comes from the U.S. Office Of Education: "Children with special learning disabilities exhibit a disorder in one or more of the basic psychological processes involved in understanding or in using spoken or written language. These may be manifested in disorders of listening, thinking, talking, reading, writing, spelling, or arithmetic. They include conditions which have been referred to as perceptual handicap, brain injury, minimal brain dysfunction, dyslexia, developmental aphasia, et cetera. They do not include learning problems which are due primarily to visual, hearing, or motor handicaps, to mental retardation, emotional disturbance or to environmental disadvantage."

2

Etiology

There are several established causes of learning disabilities. A very important factor is that of failure to organize the right and left hemispheres of the brain by not going through the crawling phase of development; this generally is six months to a year old. Some parents attempt to make things easier on themselves by placing a child in a playpen, high chair, or walker and leaving them there for hours at a time. This is supposed to free the harried housewife and mother so she can get other things done without a baby under foot. She may make things easier for herself for the moment, but there is a good chance she has contributed to the making of a learning disabled child. It is of paramount importance to have a child go through a crawling stage. This is absolutely necessary for the proper neurologic patterning that normal development demands. The average infant will discover interesting things to investigate in his or her surroundings and will make every effort to reach that which is attractive. The moment the infant starts crawling, the process of organization goes into high gear and continues right through to the next stage—that of pulling himself up to a standing position. This he will do *when he is ready*, and he should *not* be forced to stand or walk one moment sooner.[12]

One very important part of the crawling or creeping period is that of how it is done. The parent must be watchful and make sure that the "cross-crawl" pattern is used. If the left knee and the right hand go forward together, and then the right knee and the left hand

7

go forward together, there is nothing to be concerned about. This is the beginning of hemispheric organization and probably will continue right on schedule. If, however, the two left limbs and the two right limbs operate together, a problem is in the making. Care should be taken to guide the baby, actually placing the hands and knees in proper position, gently, of course.

If it is found that the child resists the correction, perhaps the patterning exercise will be of help. This is easy to do and can be made into a fun time. Lay the baby on his back, with a person on each side. The procedure is similar to crawling. One of the child's arms is carried upward over his head. The opposite knee is brought toward the abdomen simultaneously. When these limbs are returned, the opposite members are flexed and then returned. A slow, methodical rhythm is maintained for a few minutes, making sure that the proper sequence is carried out. Incorrectly done, this procedure can do more harm than good. If the person doing this has the tendency to mix up his own right and left hands, it might be better to substitute someone without that problem. This exercise must be rhythmic and must be done correctly each time.

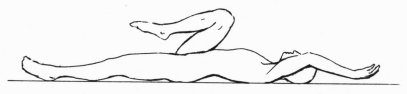

The cross-crawl

After a few sessions, it would be time to put the child on his own. Very often just a couple of days provide the correction.

If the improper crawl persists, there is probably some other structural or neurologic failure, and professional help should be sought, preferably kinesiological. Anything other than kinesiological will be more in the nature of patterning and learning by rote. Structural and neurologic correction would not be accomplished unless motion studies are done and the appropriate changes made.

*   *   *

Physical trauma, of course, must not be overlooked as a causative factor. Everytime a person meets up with his environment or the reverse, there is an effect. It might be minimal, it might be stronger, or it might even be disastrous. In any event, it is an effect, and a structural change will be brought about.

As a result of injuries, the cloacal reflex system is affected in the same way that a circuitry is marked with a memory of details in sharp clarity. Proper examination will bring to light whatever reflexes need correction.

Of course, injury comes in many shapes and sizes. One of the first we can suffer is at the time of our birth. Instruments are used, hands can be careless, labor is hurried or delayed to fit convenience. The least damage to the baby would result from cesarean section. If the mother doesn't mind the abdominal surgery and the additional cost, she might prefer to go that way. On the other side of the coin, although overall maternity mortality is extremely uncommon (9.9 deaths per 100,000 births in 1978), cesarean birth carries two to four times the risk for mortality when compared with vaginal delivery. Some maternal mortality is related to maternal illness rather than to the surgery. Cesarean birth is a major surgical procedure with morbidity greater than by vaginal delivery. Infections constitute the greatest proportion of this morbidity. The most common infections are endometritis and urinary tract and wound infections.[13]

Although less damage may result from the cesarean section, two major deficiencies take place. The birth process is a natural occurrence and, if proceeded with properly and with the aid of gravity and in a position where the mother can bear down easily to push the baby out, very little damage, if any, is done. The squat or semi-squat stance is best for this.

The normal compression and rubbing done by the mother as the baby passes through the birth canal stimulates the various neurologic processes related to the glands, helps loosen the mucus in the air passages and bowel, and gives neurologic direction to the skin. This is important in neural organization. We have all heard of being rubbed the wrong way! This is a physiological fact: we *can* be rubbed the wrong way, creating neurologic deficit.

Skin has a neurologic direction which was acquired through the birth process. A breech birth usually produces confused direction, and cesarean birth has no innate direction. In that case the direction generally will be acquired as the child matures.

At times the skin direction needs to be tested and corrected. There are various reasons for this, one of which is following surgery, which many times disturbs the skin reflexes. Plastic repair and scars are good examples of this phenomenon. This sends aberrant impulses into the central nervous system, causing symptomatology and/or neural disorganization, even in a distant part.

Later on, there is a variety of traumatic experiences, such as falls, strains, blows, even physical abuse. All of these factors go toward producing aberrations, both mental and physical. Any blow to the head, whether it be a punch, a shove, or a slap, can result in damage. The face, with fourteen bones, and the skull, with eight, are particularly vulnerable to displacement, especially in youngsters. Those most likely to be disturbed are the sphenoid, temporal, palatine, and occipital bones. The minute degrees of motion are crucial to preserving a state of normalcy. The sphenoid can become tipped, the occipital can sideslip, the palatine can become sharply arched. All of them can evidence fixation to some degree. Suffice it to say that any trauma to the head has a seriousness attached to it. There will be a price, small or large, but necessarily a price.

As the individual progresses to the walking, running, and jumping stages, another danger lurks—that of jarring. A sit-down fall or a jump from any height can result in injury quite easily. Comparatively, the head is remarkably heavy, so when the rest of the body comes to a sudden stop, the tendency of the head is to continue. It should be easy to see the potential hazard. The weight of the head is the main factor in producing injury in whiplash type accidents in the same way.

*   *   *

There is a type of injury that does not come to mind as readily as others; it is of a neurologic nature. One might ask how a neurologic effect can displace bones. If one has experienced a horrible accident, crushing news from a loved one, or some similar occurrence, has not the digestion, heart action, or breathing mechanism been affected? To some, a violent argument will be followed by diarrhea; being told of a family loss can result in instant migraine; anticipation of some important event can produce rapid pulse, breathlessness, perhaps fever. Some unfortunates suffer all three. It may be seen now that muscles are involved in all of the above events. One of the main functions of muscles is to keep bones where they belong, so the moment a muscle group weakens or goes into spasm, displacement is bound to take place.

An unnatural, displeasing, dangerous, or disgusting situation or substance, if seen, heard, touched, or tasted, can produce instantaneous muscle weakness. Of course, the body is possessed of miraculous healing powers; it can acclimate itself to many adverse circumstances and, in most instances, can shake them off rather readily. This is true if the state of bodily resistance is at par level and if the harmful occurrence isn't repeated over and over. No organism can tolerate this without evidencing the effects suffered. A good example of this is a case that comes to mind from the author's files. An eleven-year-old girl had been removed from her home by Children's Court and placed with a foster family. A short time later she was returned to her mother, only to be removed a second time and finally removed for a third time. The court was so preoccupied in attempting to preserve the status quo in the child's home, it didn't take note of the fact that an accumulation of neurologic shock was building up.

The mother's chief occupation was the entertaining of men in the house—many men—and when the traffic got too heavy, the child was recruited to help out. As a result of these repeated attacks on her psyche, she became a full-fledged dyslexic no longer knowing the difference between right and wrong or right and left, and she finally wound up failing every subject in school. Her I.Q. dropped to an ignoble twenty.

Kinesiology, in this instance, corrected the positive findings; the outlook has changed to cheerful and smiling and the I.Q. rocketed up to ninety in three weeks of treatment. If this child can be given the chance of leading a normal life, her problems with learning mechanisms will evaporate and her skills will return to what they had been.

*   *   *

The next effect we must look at is that of adverse chemistry. The total organism is fed and nurtured through biochemistry. The food that we see and like and wish to eat will look to *us* like steaks and chops, fruits and vegetables, butter, starch and sweets. The digestive system sees the food differently. It looks these things over, grinds them up, adds a few digestive enzymes, throws some bile into the pot, stirs for a while, absorbs what it thinks the body needs, and discards the rest. During that process the conglomeration was just a happy mixture of proteins, fats, carbohydrates, vitamins, and minerals—sort of a sophisticated chemistry set.

If some of this chemistry proves to be wrong for the body, there will be a reaction—anywhere from mild to violent. Again the body is capable of weathering occasional lapses, but constant repetition of the wrong ingredients will bring down the walls of Jericho and the wrath of judgment.

Let's take one item for an example—sugar. The central nervous system needs the equivalent of two teaspoons of sugar per twenty-four hours; anything more than that is not food. More than that counts up very rapidly. A wedge of apple pie and a ball of ice cream is the equivalent of about twenty-two teaspoons of sugar! There are about nine teaspoons in a can of soda! The average person now consumes about 200 pounds of sugar per year! Our grandparents used less than seventy pounds. By 1969, this had risen to one hundred and four (*CF*).

Sugar is only one of many substances that have a deleterious effect on the organism; others are caffeine, chocolate, nicotine, dyes, bleaches, preservatives, flavorings, seasonings, and the whole gamut of artificialities that the human is subjected to. "Human" is used here purposely because animal husbandry has known for many years how important nutrition is to the qualities of performance, appearance, vitality, longevity, and breeding capabilities. Why has all of this been overlooked in the care and feeding of *homo sapiens*?

Could it be possible that the eternal chase for the almighty dollar has clouded our vision?

In reality, if the synthetic ingredients were left out of the food basket, we would discover the true, natural taste of things which has been removed by all the refining, adding, and subtracting. Who has not had the opportunity of comparing an organically grown tomato or carrot with those produced in a greenhouse and fertilized with chemicals? The first looks, tastes, and smells like food, the second like cardboard. But, what is more important, the first is rich in minerals, vitamins, and nutritional value; the second is artificial, artfully produced to be all one color, all one size, all one weight— like they had been turned out with a cookie cutter on a workbench. It is more profitable to have them all fit in the same-sized box or package.

Regarding the stresses of the adolescent, one takes cognizance of the fact that nutritional imbalances are often quite visible in poor skin condition, brittle and lusterless hair, poor muscle tone, uneven strength and coordination, lack of physical stamina, and excess poundage.[25] Youth in the United States face a dim future in terms of physical prowess and mental well-being. The stark contrast between high nutrient demand in their lives and low nutrient delivery in their diets should be a matter of concern and action for parents and institutional administrators.[26]

Muscle tone will never respond healthfully with that kind of nutrition; and balanced muscle tone is necessary to maintain skeletal integrity. If there are neuro-musculoskeletal imbalances, anything can go wrong. Among the possibilities are cranial-facial displacements which, in proper combination, can result in learning disabilities. The importance of proper nutritional balance cannot be overemphasized. In a study of preschool children in Chile, tests for motor, language, adaptive, and personal-social skills were made. Children scoring lowest in all areas were also those who were most malnourished (Monckeberg, 1968).[25]

Regarding children, fetal alcohol syndrome (FAS) is an established consequence of alcohol consumption by the pregnant mother. These children are often mentally retarded as a result of prenatal alcohol exposure. Some may not suffer such immediately obvious effects but later display hyperactivity and severe, persistent learning problems (Shaywitz, 1980).[25]*

*   *   *

Finally, we reach the well-meant but wrongful propensity of some people who attempt to determine for their children whether they should be left-handed or right-handed. During the organizational stage, right or left dominance is decided, regardless of our wishes. Everything neurologic is both predicated upon this fact and developed by this fact. It is most important in the successful utilization of the centering mechanism of the body. Propagation in the animal world would be virtually impossible without it. Far too many parents, and let's not forget the grandparents, attempt to influence the child's dominance, realizing of course that the world around us is basically right-handed. Therefore, it should follow that all children should be right-handed, right? Wrong! The future neurologic welfare of the individual depends on proper development, and forcing dominance on a child can result in many forms and degrees of organizational disabling.

There are other ways of producing the same or similar effect. One girl became disabled because algebra was forced upon her in high school. Her mathematics gave her no trouble until she started battling with x plus y equals z. It boggled her mind, which, no doubt, had two strikes against it to begin with. Her dietary indiscretions were many. According to the patient's statement, the assault of algebra upon her robbed her of any ability she might have had with arithmetic.

With a minimal amount of kinesiological treatment this case was resolved. The diet was regulated and the structural corrections made. After a little brushing up on her arithmetic, the lady straightened out readily.

There are many instances of people having a situation forced upon them wherein they are unable to cope. Particularly strong

*Courtesy of Joseph D. Beasley, M.D., in *The Impact of Nutrition on the Health of Americans*. Medicine and Nutrition Project, sponsored by the Bard College Center.

frustration is extremely difficult to handle. It can affect us physiologically to the point of actual illness, and an end result may be a structural misalignment, which, in turn, creates further problems with the nervous system and circulation.

Another patient, an eleven-year-old boy with the same history, that of being urged to switch to right-handedness, was brought into the office. His father, while acting as soccer and baseball coach, realized that not only had the boy consistently stayed in the background during soccer practice and games, he had *never gotten* a hit while up at bat during baseball practice. After only *one* treatment, following a kinesiological survey, not only did Gary go out and become the star of the soccer team, he also got two hits out of four times at bat in the very next game in which he played.

His first words afterward were that it was the first time he had actually been able to tell where the ball was. Tests had shown the lateral eye muscle fibers of the right eye and the medial ones of the left eye to be in spasm. This made it very difficult for him to bat successfully because of the acute strain of attempting to look to his left accurately. This would cause a deficit in the normal neural rhythm, the interruption of which would bring about confusion in the muscle coordination system. This would result in the boy missing the ball. When the spasm was removed, he was able to swing his eyes readily to the left.

Gary's problem on the soccer field was somewhat similar. He found himself able to kick successfully if the ball came at him from his right but was dismayed to find that a ball on his left went past him because of his inability to focus his eyes in that direction. Nobody seemed to notice that his difficulty was only one-sided. His playing was seen to be erratic, connecting at times and missing at times, so it didn't take long for him to absent himself from the spotlight for fear of what he saw as stupid failure. It made him appear clumsy, and what eleven-year-old can take that?

He now looks forward to his practice sessions and games, and his parents are enraptured.

3

Structural Abnormalities

There is a fact which bears repeating. There are several structures which, if misaligned or misplaced, can be blamed for learning disabilities. There are bones such as the sphenoid, temporal, palatine, and occiput. There are the temporal-mandibular joints and all the sutures between the cranial bones. Considering that there are twenty-two bones altogether in the skull and face, it is no small wonder that several combinations of structural abnormality are possible. The sphenoid can be tilted, the occiput sideslipped, the palatine overly arched, the temporal, parietal, or frontal jammed. Present research has determined that with three or more of these cranial faults plus a temporal fault, the patient is a dyslexic. With less than these, the case is only that of simple learning disability.[24]

One may ask, "How does the displacement of these bones cause neurological problems?" It is quite simple really. Unequal pressure areas are created on the contents of the cranial vault. The central nervous system is reaching out constantly to "test the wind," so to speak. It is concerned with the positioning of, the action of, the response of every single part and is quick to notice an abnormality. The result is immediate and dramatic. Muscle tone weakens, blood circulation is affected, sensitivity is changed, secretions are increased or decreased. Fluid pressures in the tissues are altered. Even the blood pressure goes up or down.

The excitement is at a very high pitch when, following an almost infinitesimal bony manipulation, the above symptoms disappear. It

16

is a nonforce procedure which is easily borne by infants as well as children and adults. It is noninvasive, nonchemical, and nonsurgical. Nothing is removed, nothing is added. The patient is the same as before but with the abnormalities corrected.

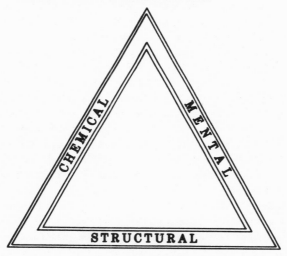

The Triad of Health

By interrelating the factors of the triad of health, i.e., mental, chemical, structural, it should readily be understood how dependent each is upon the others.

1. Adverse chemistry can alert the bodily forces to bring about rapid repair, but if the effect is too strong, the structural and mental sides become involved. There can be changes in the skeletal balance due to muscular weakness or spasm, and there can occur as well changes within the neurologic system.

2. "Psychosomatic" really needs no explaining. The influence of the nervous system over the structure and the chemical economy is direct and immediate. No organ will function properly unless the nervous system is intact. Digestive enzymes are disturbed, muscle tone is altered, thereby creating stress on the skeletal components.

The bony structures are adversely affected by improper nutrition. Many adults, when reaching ages forty and up, can evidence signs of osteoporosis. This is due to a paucity of minerals in the diet and can result in fracture. Another important reaction is the abnormal torque of various bones, in particular, that of the sphenoid. The proper action of this segment of the skull is paramount to mental stability and is one of the main factors in treating the learning disabled. The degree of normalcy of the nervous system also can affect the posture. Most mental aberrations result in the hang-dog look, the woe-is-me syndrome—head forward, dorsal area kyphotic, belly distended, feet dragging.

The gracilis and sartorius muscles are important in the action of the pelvis. These muscles are weakened if the adrenal glands become hyperactive. This is an excellent example of the mental and chemical sides of the triad affecting the third or structural side.

3. The structural side of the triad is just as important when it is seen that the mental and chemical are affected just as readily in that direction. An example would be the bruising of the sole of the foot. How on earth could this have any connection with the neurologic or chemical aspects of the body, one could ask. Again it is quite simple. There would be the almost immediate development of a limp, leading to a distortion of the pelvis. This would impart a stress on the gracilis and sartorius muscles, which in turn would affect the adrenal glands neurologically. As well, the proprioceptors would be improperly stimulated by the awkwardness of gait, which would place stress on the occipital area. The next stage could be headaches, leading to cranial faults—a perfect start for the learning disabled syndrome. Almost any structural abnormality has a direct or indirect effect on the mental and/or chemical function. They can stress, they can poison, they can stimulate, they can inhibit. No neurological or chemical action will be at par value while there is a structural imbalance sufficient to cause interference. One such abnormality is brought about by wearing high heels. There is a gross physiological disorientation brought about which causes great stress and leads to switching—a breakdown of normal brain hemisphere symmetry.[8] This subject will be more fully covered in a later chapter.

4

Education

Earlier in this text it was stated that, although magnificent strides have been made in working with children with learning disabilities, there was something lacking. This was in no way meant to be derogatory. The many teachers and planners are to be praised, not only for their abilities but also for their dedication. What has been lacking is the knowledge that there are many of these children with slight structural faults, not physically noticeable, which have been brought about by neurologic, chemical, or physical injury. No amount of drilling in the three Rs is going to do the whole job until or unless these structural faults are discovered and corrected. The procedure is painless, quick, and all accomplished by hand.

The educators have worked long and hard in ferreting out the disabled from the student population in order to enter them into special remedial classes. The children are tested, and, when found lacking in memory, reading comprehension, or mathematics skills, it is presumed that they are dyslexic, borderline, or somewhere in between. This designation usually remains tagged to the student as long as he or she is in the school system. If items are taught but not comprehended or remembered, there is no reason for the child to be any smarter in them subsequent to kinesiological treatment than he was before. What he *will* have is the ability to absorb new material like the proverbial sponge. His comprehension, memory, agility, reading, and mathematics will show tremendous gain almost immediately. The remedial part of his training would have to be continued in order for him to catch up with the things he passed over while disabled.

It goes without saying that the treatment must be done correctly for it to be effective and lasting. The cloacal reflexes must be negative; the occiput must sit straight and solid upon the atlas, the first vertebra of the spine. The cranial segments must have free motion so the respiratory mechanism operates unimpeded, and they also must be balanced. The hemispheric organization must be established and dominance determined. The right brain deals with the emotional aspect of understanding, the appreciation of art, music, crafts, colors, and nature. The left brain carries the logical, practical, mathematical responsibilities. It is important that the two sides carry on their appointed tasks, and when this doesn't happen, there is good possibility that neurologic switching has taken place. This fact, along with various cranial faults, points to the person with a learning disability.

The very first moment a child is judged, by testing, to have a learning impairment, he or she should have the consultation of a kinesiologist specializing in the various facets of learning disability. The doctor will carry the patient through the survey accurately, will lay out a course of action with nutritional guidance, will prescribe any corrective exercises necessary, and will negate all neurologic faults that are correctable.

For the child whose disability takes him through the miseries of dyslexia, some of his worst experiences are met while trying to learn to read, write, use numbers, and, above all else, be able to comprehend vocal instruction. The interpretation of the information coming into the consciousness is inconsistent; a particular letter, word, or symbol is sometimes altered, reversed, or interchanged. The "furry cat" might be *tac* or *atc*. What possible sense can the child make out of "furry atc" or the "furry tac"? He will squint his eyes, giving rise to the thought of a visual problem, or perhaps ask that it be repeated, suggesting that he may be suffering from a hearing loss. In the meantime, the child has slid past one more word, term, or situation that he can't comprehend and can add that to the pile of bypassed learning he is accumulating. The rest of the students know what a cat is and can use the word properly at all times for the rest of their lives. Our hapless dyslexic, who does not know what a *tac* or an *atc* is, will probably shrug it off, cry secretly, or perhaps act up in order to cover up. The more the child tries to make sense of what he's looking at or hearing, the more tense he becomes and the more the word changes and moves about.

Scanning lines while reading is another very large problem. Following from one line to the next, the dyslexics may skip one or more lines when returning their eyes to the left, Many times they cannot follow the same line across the page. Not only does this lead to frustration but also to restlessness. They want the reading lesson over with so they possibly can relax with something else—anything else but that "dumb reading." Of course, if math comes next, they are again in a dilemma. As was pointed out earlier, the addition (+) and the multiplication (×) symbols are exactly the same shape and size and one becomes the other just with a small tilt. The subtraction (−) and division (÷) symbols are, again, quite similar. The disabled can "think" the two dots or leave them out—whichever the optic nerve has conveyed to the brain.

One important reason for the inability to recognize the addition, multiplication, subtraction, and division symbols is that many dyslexics suffer from nystagmus, a rapid eye movement, usually from side to side. This condition may be caused by extra stress on the imbalanced or spastic eye muscles when they are forced to move from one side to the other in normal reading procedure or when attempting to concentrate or focus on a particular spot. Obviously this will cause the letters to move about and change position. It can cause the addition and multiplication signs to move or seem to rotate and therefore become indistinguishable.

Because vowels usually are confused and/or not distinguishable, many words are not understood, and the dyslexic often will ask, "What do you mean by that?", sometimes to the most casual statement. This striving to understand what is being said often leads to impatience and perhaps even anger on the part of the speaker, be he parent, friend, or teacher.

The dyslexic has learned early on not to ask, "What did you say?" or "Please repeat that," because if the speaker uses the same words again, there will be no better understanding than there was at first. The next ploy is for the disabled to ask that a word be defined, on the chance that a synonym will be used which he hopes he will recognize.

Unfortunately, there is no consistency; the child sees and hears almost any variety of combined forms and makes out of them whatever he is able. He has to invent ways of masking his short-comings any way he can. He can't handle the extreme frustration and many times finds himself embroiled with his peers, parents, teachers, or even the law.

Many a parent will feel so badly for the faltering child that he or she will cover the lack by helping dishonestly. This misplaced kind-ness can't make much difference while the son or daughter is in class, however. Better by far to cooperate with the educational factors and help legitimately. A good example of misguided parental help is the student who can't read very well but can memorize verbatim anything he hears. He will listen to another child's recitation, carry it home to his mother word for word, and then she, in just another head-in-the-sand maneuver, will put the material in her child's notebook. She has, again, covered up his discrepancy instead of coming to grips with the facts—her child is disabled and needs help of a specific nature, not that of being able to lean on everyone else for his entire scholastic career.

Reading is a very natural task for the average child to accomplish. He or she is led into the art slowly, being taught by sounds, pictures, toys, songs, and other varieties of learning materials. There is no great effort expended in most cases. Reading starts off being a really fun thing to do and hopefully will remain firm in later years. The disabled is another story. He meets up with several problems. If he reads to himself, not holding the book, he comprehends a small degree of the contents. If the book is picked up and held while reading, a lesser amount is understood because the brain is stressed by two things to do at once. There is more confusion and much embarrassment, which lead to nervous tension, hence poorer per-formance. If this same child holds the book and reads out loud, he is attempting three things at once—reading, speaking, and holding. Often this is just too much coordination to handle.

There are many degrees of performance in those with dyslexia. Some can do more than others, different combinations of tasks than others, and even in the same person, the abilities vary from day to day.

Strong motivation from within and a whole lot of help from without will help the learning process. If the child becomes interested in a story or project, can relate to it, can picture it, there is a good chance he will stick to it and gradually make some sense out of it. He will then go on, relating to other things, learning to read, write, do mathematics, et cetera. Hardly ever will this be entirely normal comprehension; he will rarely be totally sure of things. He will perform at an almost normal level ultimately and, with the exception of spelling (all the right letters but not always in the right order), can get lost in the crowd so that, hopefully, very few others will be aware of the disability.

He will avoid playing word games such as Scrabble for fear of being exposed to people unaware of his problem. No amount of training or special tutoring will transform a dyslexic into a nondyslexic. The neurology must be unscrambled, organized, and made operative. When and if this is accomplished, the condition is neutralized, and the baby, child, or adult becomes like any other of the surrounding peers.

Most researchers today believe that special tutoring and special teaching techniques are the only answer to the learning problem. Fortunately, there is much benefit to this, provided the dyslexic is recognized as such by parent or teacher and that an active role is taken in the learning process. In many cases this does not happen, and because most children experience some confusion in the initial stages of letter and number appreciation, the testing procedures are not instituted until the third grade. By this time many bad habits are established and traits become ingrained—frustration, lack of self-esteem, knowing there is a difference, accepting the appellations of "stupid" and "lazy." Some become disciplinary problems and there is much to undo.

Many get so used to the problem that they lose the initiative to better themselves. They tend to believe they are just dumb, stupid, lazy, clumsy, inept, sloppy, and disoriented, getting lost going around the corner. And you can be sure their peers are going to apply the name calling in a steady stream.

They accept this as a fact of life and never try to overcome the disability because when they try, they fail. They don't seek help because they don't even know they have the disability. They learn to lean on mother and father figures who always seem to be available for help in straightening things out for them. They get along by doing the best they can under very trying circumstances.

One of the problems until now has been the inaccuracy, confusion, and diversity of testing procedures. There have been no definitive, standardized neurologic tests because dyslexia is a condition and not a disease. There have been certain eye tests promulgated, but these too are not definitive. In most cases the parents run the gamut from doctor to doctor, from institution to institution, ad infinitum, running into the expenditure of many thousands of dollars, only to be told that although there is nothing really wrong with the child, he can't read, write, or talk properly and doesn't walk or run with facility.

Some school districts have a corps of special teachers who run remedial classes for these troubled children. Many don't, however, provide special programs for this type of student. Considering the large proportion of learning disabled in this country, we are dealing with a staggering number needing help.

The special training and teaching techniques geared for these unfortunate people work well, although the person still has the disability and life is, at best, difficult in a world of words, signs, maps, warnings, et cetera.

Some pediatricians assure the parents that the children are asymptomatic, just "slow learners," and will grow out of the imagined problem. They point out that there are many children with similar sluggishness and they have no need to worry. In the meantime, the poor child slides into the ignominious category of "dyslexic." This same pediatrician loses contact with the child as he grows older, and, therefore, he assumes the child outgrew the problem as he said he would.

Unless the parents are persistent, the child is fated for a miserable school experience, perhaps dropping out, perhaps running away, perhaps becoming a burden to himself, his parents, or society in general. He can't cope, he is ashamed of his inability to read, write or do simple mathematics, so he doesn't seek help and ends up in a lower stratum of society.

There are exceptions who attain academic or job success, go into the professions, or otherwise reach their objectives. This is with great personal sacrifice, special learning and performance tricks, and much perseverance. However, for every one who fights his way to the top, there are thousands who never do.

Up to now, even though these people learn to cope with their hardship and seem to have overcome its difficulties, they still have all the problems associated with the condition, and, therefore, the quality of their lives is lessened. In most cases they live in fear that others will find out and therefore think less of them. They don't read newspapers and they shy away from restaurants—they can't read the menu. They avoid involvement in serious conversations because they find it difficult to follow the thought, and they generally live on the edge of everything.

There was an executive with a major company who would take his reports and other business papers home with him each evening. He would spend hours memorizing them so he could appear to have a thorough grip on his affairs the next day. His social life didn't amount to much. He didn't have the time. He was much too busy attending to his intellectual emergency. His place on the board would be shortlived if the truth were known. There wouldn't be a great deal of trust placed in a man who could hear one thing and do another, or perhaps read a list of specifications of great importance to the company and wind up ordering three carloads of widgets when the need was really for three gross of diwgets.

His lot, during his corporate career, would be to devote every spare moment repeating over and over, literally carving grooves into his kaleidoscopic brain so as to aid him in retaining a good amount of that for which his job has made him responsible.

There is a good chance that, with very little effort, his problem can be minimized, if not cleared up entirely, by kinesiological survey.

5

Findings

The child with a learning disability is attempting to cope with a world much too big for him. It is too fast and too smart, given to great facility and normal coordination. A number of these children are left-handed, and there are also quite a few who tried to be left-handed but were discouraged along the way. This, as we have seen, can lead to neurologic confusion.

They seem, a good deal of the time, to be carrying out instructions opposite to what is wanted. This, in the learning disabled, is not disobedience. They are seen as having a behavioral problem when, in reality, they are doing the best they can to please, if only to avoid discipline.

Much unpleasantness could be avoided if the parents would understand the simple fact that, in these cases, "performance is in the eye of the performer." The child sees himself doing exactly what he was asked to do when, in truth, he is doing the opposite.

During the organizational phase of the infant, many times right or left dominance does not take place. This starts the child off in a mixed or perhaps ambidextrous pattern.

One mother put it rather interestingly. She said her son was not ambidextrous but rather ambi-nondextrous and indicated no real coordination with either hand. Of course, there are exceptions to this; we find some of these children with an uncanny ability to put things together or take them apart. However, for the most part, dyslexic children cannot tie their shoes, button their jackets or shirts, or buckle a belt. If, by chance, some can, it is with great difficulty.

Finding a high percentage of the disabled with left-handedness would seem to indicate a right brain dominance when it is generally accepted that the left brain is the logical, thinking mathematical hemisphere. Oftentimes if one side is preferred, there still is a mixed dominance tendency, such as right hand and left foot, right eye and left ear.

Sometimes the mixed dominance doesn't make too much difference; either can be used, but it still remains true that many of the disabled use one or the other without knowing which is which. When it becomes important, there must be some key worked out, for instance, the dancer on stage who *must* know, so she uses the audience as her "right" and the backdrop as her "left."

Rather than go through life making constant apology for ineptness, many dyslexics abandon reading and writing and point themselves in other directions. They try to take up vocations which are not demanding in the areas of their weaknesses. Through perseverance, practice, and determination, some of them really excel. There are sports champions, financiers, scientists, and engineers who have bubbled right to the top of their chosen careers—but don't ask them to read a book or find their way to an unknown location.

There are women who are fair homemakers as long as they don't have to go shopping (can't add money) or do any sewing (can't thread a needle). There are athletes who excel in their sport but can't sign for their paychecks. There are social lions who are much sought after by perennial hostesses—but don't ask them to play bridge; they wouldn't know a spade from a snow shovel.

The following is a case in point. In discussing a chosen occupation with a prospective patient, he stated, "Doc, I have to make a living. I can't read, can't write, and can't do math, so I can't get an office job. I can't be a mechanic because of handling small tools. I can't put a screw into a small hole. I don't know which way to turn the screwdriver or twist the wrench. I can't be an electrician for most of the same reasons, and there is no way I can handle live wires. I can't be a plumber because I don't know which way to turn the pipe or fittings, and forget it if I'm upside down under a sink or something. I wouldn't know which way anything goes—so, I've become a carpenter. As long as you're not in a hurry and I don't have to use power saws, I'll get the job done even though I miss the nail a lot!''

What a commentary on how things should have been for this man. In his days in school (a one-room schoolhouse in a southern, mountain state), not too much was known about helping him. In all probability, he was several years old before anyone realized that anything more was amiss perhaps than a sluggishness in his comprehension and dexterity. By this time, his peers had gone on without him, that is, those who didn't have a similar problem.

In examining statistics, one finds that eighty percent of jail inmates are unable to read. If this fact is followed to a conclusion, we can draw a bead on one of the major reasons for such a large penal population. Do we stick with our twenty percent of these people being dyslexic? That is probably a very optimistic figure. Considering that learning disabilities contribute to so much frustration and poor performance, it is more likely a much higher percentage with the institutionalized. They have struggled like everyone else but few have succeeded. This certainly opens the door to brushes with the law in various areas, hence an overcrowded jail. As a matter of fact, if kinesiology were investigated with an eye to screening inmates, there would be a very good chance of rehabilitation being more successful than it is at present.

Howard E. Rome, M.D., senior consultant in psychiatry at the Mayo Clinic, stated: "There is a body of cumulative evidence which holds that a significant number of juvenile delinquents have reading problems."

Several years ago an exciting statistic was read into the *Congressional Record* (*CR*). Chiropractic manipulation was put to the test on an experimental basis in a sanitarium for the mentally retarded. Everyone was astounded to discover that twenty-eight percent of these people returned to living a normal life as a result. Spinal and cranial balancing were done, much the same as that which has been done for so many years at Spears Chiropractic Hospital (*SP*) in Denver. Also, the Spears family pioneered skull molding, and the third generation is now hard at work solving the many problems thrown at them from all over the world (*SP*).

One very obvious finding among many is that by restoring the structural, neurologic, and chemical integrity to the present and future of our kids, we will be protecting them from the possibilities of learning disabilities, with the concomitant hazards of frustration, hyperkinesis, lack of intellectual prowess, and the potential of lawlessness. If a child has the proper beginnings he or she is entitled to, there is a very good chance that the better things in life will be made available. What better way to develop into a solid citizen?

In some instances, a dyslexic will falter, lose ground momentarily, or fail completely. One such case was that of a twenty-three-year-old man who had a nasty virus attack that caused him to lose all the improvement he had gained. This was shortlived, however, because as soon as the virility of the illness abated, the advance of facility returned to what it had been.

Another child had a rather nasty domestic problem arise at home. This, too, had the effect of robbing the patient of most of the plus values he had shown. When the family matter finally was resolved, all went well with the child.

Occasionally, the doctor runs into a personality trait that no amount of correction can get through. The person or child is thoroughly convinced that nothing much has ever been done to help, and he or she is equally sure that anything done now is just a waste of time. There can be actual belligerence. Unless the negativity can be breached, there is almost a certainty that the treatment will be to little avail, if any at all.

One case history is the account of a male child who, in addition to being a dyslexic, also had some rather bad allergic responses from time to time. At a point well into the procedure for his learning disability, he had a nasty allergy attack. While the period of distress lasted—about thirty-six hours—it was as if no improvement had ever occurred. As soon as his body overcame the allergenic episode, better than ninety percent of his forward progress returned all on its own. This certainly points to the hookup between physiology and neurology in these conditions. If the neural part of the triad of health is made to falter by unbalanced physiology; if the reverse occurs, where the body manages to circumvent the mental processes, the state of well-being is disturbed, symptoms begin to appear, and there is a whole package of health problems possible.

One of the discouraging outcomes in treating dyslexia is that of having a patient disappointed because he hasn't become a good reader or mathematician instantly. The patient had leaned on his kinesiological correction as being a cure-all for his hodgepodge of intellectual failings; what he has not accepted, and this oftentimes is part of the main problem, is that while he was in remedial classes, his own peers were going along at normal pace and, of course, leaving him behind more and more. By removing his neurologic blockage, balancing the frame, and correcting the nutritional habits, the stage has been set for him to be *receptive* to *learning*; the learning or drilling or practicing is now up to his teachers and himself. His equipment is in order and can now be programmed. Practice is the key to all successful retention, so it is paramount to continue remedial training. Only in this way can the learning disabled take his or her place in the normal scheme of things.

If there were any doubt of this, consider for a moment the musician. Can any meaningful success be derived without practice on a regular basis? Without the means to learn, without the repetition of practice, and without the dedication of thoroughgoing teachers, no one will prosper in the skills to which he directs himself.

6

Case Histories

The following charts have been taken from the authors' files with a small degree of choice—that of selecting with an eye to a proper mix of age, sex, dominance, and major weaknesses. Attention is called to the turning point in each case, marking the reversal in the condition. An attempt has been made to offer variety in the cases so it may be appreciated that every situation differs from all others.

Dyslexia certainly has no respect for caste or stratum. It can happen to anyone who has neurologic, physical, or chemical trauma, as well as genetic inheritance. The good part is that virtually all who are so disabled can have the condition relieved.

The reader.will note that the first findings are at the time of the first examination; the second column shows the results of the first treatment; the third shows those of the second treatment. The single asterisk denotes the turning point in each item of testing; the double asterisk points to complete clearance of the item. In most cases, the cessation and clearance of these findings is the first such experience the patient has had in his or her whole life.

CASE #1: Anthony   Age 7 months   Male

Born

8-10-81, Jamaica, New York, Mary Immaculate Hospital. Admitted to Flushing Hospital, New York, on 3-30-82 with multiple epileptic seizures in both waking and sleeping phases.

31

History

Amniocentesis performed; blood was discovered in specimen. Immediate cesarean section was ordered.

Findings

Pilonidal cyst. Parents were advised to remove by surgery at two years of age.

Hospitalization

Baby admitted seven months of age with seizures several times daily.

Medication

Phenobarbital, Dilantin, Depakene

Prognosis

"Perhaps will grow out of it in twelve years."

Symptoms

Refusal to crawl or show interest in surroundings

Diagnosis

Brain damage

Notes on Case #1, Anthony: Baby was examined by kinesiological survey. The technique of spheno-basilar lift was decided upon, on the basis of research by Drs. Major DeJarnette and George Goodheart. The primary state of interference in infants is that of a respiratory fault, and the testing is done using the parent as a surrogate factor.

Outcome: two weeks of treatment (spheno-basilar lift only) resulted in complete clearance of all symptomatology. He started crawling immediately and took an active interest in people and things around him. At present writing, baby is almost two and a half years old. He has not had one instance of seizure and walks and talks with total normalcy.

(Case #1 has been included not because of a learning problem or dyslexia but as a dramatic example of the effect of cranial correction which, along with the eye muscle technique described later, is the basis of the dyslexic treatment.)

CASE #2:   Gary B.   Age 11   Male

	At Exam	2nd Visit	3rd Visit
Dominance	Mixed	Mixed	Mixed
Gait	Unilateral	Unilateral	Unilateral
Shoe tying	Average	Average	Improved*
Crawling	—	—	—
Calisthenics	Poor	Good*	Excellent**
Directional instruction	Uncooperative	Good*	Excellent**

*Turning point in each test
**Clearance in each test

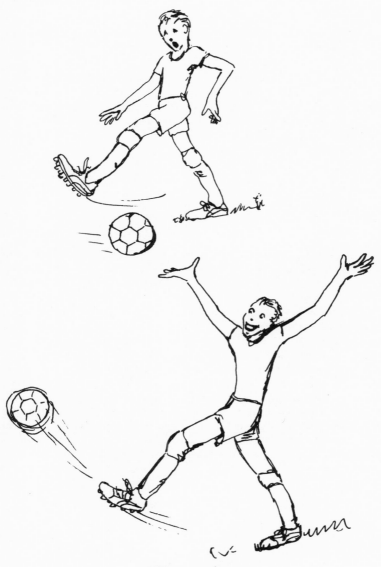

Victory at last

	At Exam	2nd Visit	3rd Visit
Muscle tone	Fair	Fair	Improved*
Mechanical ability	Good	Good	Good
Colors	Good	Good	Good
Comprehension	Fair	Good*	Excellent**
Emotions	Fair	Good*	Good
Hyperkinesis	Fair	Good*	Excellent**
Vowel pronunciation	Good	Good	Good
Reading, free	Fair	Fair	Good*
Reading, held	Poor	Fair	Good*
Reading, feet crossed	Poor	Fair	Good*
Writing	Fair	Good*	Good
Arithmetic	Fair	Good*	Excellent**
Cloacal reflexes	Several	Two*	None**
Cranial faults	Five	Three*	None**
Ocular lock	Positive	Positive	Negative**

Notes on Case #2, Gary B.: Gary responded to treatment so quickly, he gained about ninety percent of his improvement following his first session. With so many disabling items besetting him, the return to normal was nothing short of miraculous.

Gary's father is a coach and had the heartbreaking experience of watching his son hold back whenever he was called upon to play. He would hide when he should have stood up to be counted on. How could he continue to try when it always ended in failure? Now he is playing as well as anyone else on the team. His reading has improved; he has discovered a talent for drawing he never had before. He has become a model child, ready, willing, and able to join his family, teachers, and peers with interest and enthusiasm. His school psychologist has commented on the excellent change that has taken place. Gary's report card, issued in June, showed excellent improvement in social studies and spelling. He has shown marked improvement in sports, cooperation, comprehension, arithmetic, reading, drawing, and hyperkinesis. He will be reading one hour per day during the summer.

CASE #3:   *Shelley*   *Age 32*   *Female*

	At Exam	2nd Visit	3rd Visit
Dominance	Left	Left	Left
Gait	Unilateral	Unilateral	Unilateral
Shoe tying	Poor	Fair	Good*

	At Exam	2nd Visit	3rd Visit
Crawling	—	—	—
Calisthenics	Poor	Fair	Good*
Directional instruction	Fair	Fair	Good*
Muscle tone	Good	Good	Good
Mechanical ability	Poor	Fair	Good*
Colors	Good	Good	Good
Comprehension	Fair	Good*	Good
Emotions	Normal	Normal	Normal
Hyperkinesis	Negative	Negative	Negative
Vowel pronunciation	Normal	Normal	Normal
Reading, free	Fair	Fair	Good*
Reading, held	Poor	Improved*	Good**
Reading, feet crossed	Poor	Fair	Fair
Writing	Fair	Fair	Good*
Arithmetic	Poor	Good*	Excellent**
Cloacal reflexes	Five	Three	None**
Cranial faults	Four	Two	None**
Ocular lock	Positive	Negative**	Negative

Notes on Case #3, Shelley: Shelley's case was a good example of structural and neurologic trauma. She was physically abused throughout her formative years, and she suffered a great deal of mental anguish as well. At the high school level, she was forced to take algebra, which she couldn't comprehend at all because of her inability to read with understanding. Although her arithmetic had been fairly good through grammar school, the effect of the experience with algebra had driven all reasoning ability out of her head. Her arithmetic marks plummeted. It wasn't until treatment was begun that she showed improvement and it came back rapidly. Shelley's physical abilities returned as well. She had been unable to fasten a belt buckle, tie laces, catch or hit a ball, fasten buttons, or do normal sewing and ironing. All of these failures disappeared and she is elated.

CASE #4: Diane D. Age 11 Female

	At Exam	2nd Visit	3rd Visit
Dominance	Mixed	Mixed	Mixed
Gait	Contralateral	Unilateral**	Unilateral
Shoe tying	Poor	Good*	Good
Crawling	Contralateral	Unilateral**	Unilateral

	At Exam	2nd Visit	3rd Visit
Calisthenics	Sloppy	Fair	Good**
Directional instruction	Good	Good	Good
Muscle tone	Poor	Fair	Fair
Mechanical ability	Poor	Poor	Fair
Colors	Good	Good	Good
Comprehension	Fair	Good*	Good
Emotions	Good	Good	Excellent**
Hyperkinesis	Good	Good	Good
Vowel pronunciation	Good	Good	Good
Reading, free	Poor	Fair	Good*
Reading, held	Poor	Fair	Good*
Reading, feet crossed	Poor	Fair	Good*
Writing	Good	Good	Good
Arithmetic	Poor	Good*	Good
Cloacal reflexes	Four	Two*	None**
Cranial faults	Four	Three	Clear**
Ocular lock	Positive	Negative	Negative

Notes on Case #4, Diane D.: The following are three attempts at letter writing in stated sequence:

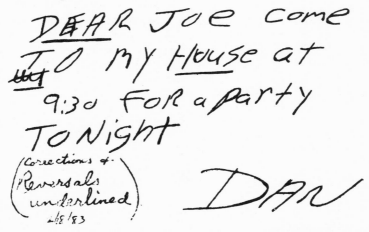

First writing test: Note the A changed to E, the U to O and the T, crossed at the bottom first and then corrected by crossing out. The signature is incomplete.

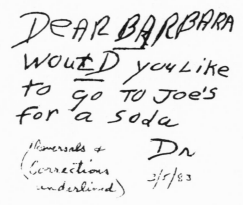

Second writing test: Note the R changed to A, the D to L, and again the signature is incomplete. This second test was done about two and a half weeks later.

Third writing test: Note the vast improvement except for the phonetic spelling of the word tonight. The signature is now complete, probably denoting the child's building of a sense of worth in herself. She is proud to say who she is. The note has better form and shows that a little care and consideration has been put into it.

Diane, when shown tests one and two, said, "I don't believe I wrote those and I don't remember doing it. They don't look nice." There is a hiatus of two and one half months between test two and test three. Diane had no treatment during this period because of a domestic problem at home. She showed marked improvement in writing, reading, comprehension, normal walking gait, emotions, social studies, and mathematics. She was discharged as clear.

CASE #5:   *Louis H.*   *Age 19*   *Male*

	At Exam	2nd Visit	3rd Visit
Dominance	Mixed	Mixed	Mixed
Gait	Unilateral	Unilateral	Unilateral
Shoe tying	—	—	—
Crawling	—	—	—
Calisthenics	Good	Good	Good
Directional instruction	Poor	Poor	Fair
Muscle tone	Good	Good	Good
Mechanical ability	Fair	Good**	Good
Colors	—	—	—
Comprehension	Poor	Poor	Good**
Emotions	Normal	Normal	Normal
Hyperkinesis	Normal	Normal	Normal
Vowel pronunciation	Good	Good	Good
Reading, free	Poor	Poor	Good**
Reading, held	Poor	Poor	Good**
Reading, legs crossed	Poor	Poor	Fair
Writing	Fair	Improved*	Improved
Arithmetic	—	—	—
Cloacal reflexes	Four	Two	None**
Cranial faults	Three	Two	None**
Ocular lock	Positive	Negative**	Negative

Notes on Case #5, Louis H.: Louis is in college. He has persevered and has had to struggle much harder than most to maintain passing grades. His special education teachers through grammar school did their very best to work with him where he needed it. Certainly he never would have reached college if they had not persevered along with him. Two of his greatest difficulties were reading and comprehending the spoken word. When his higher education courses called for lecture classes and research in the library, he felt almost totally lost. He leaned heavily upon his parents. It was the greatest thrill of his life when, following three kinesiological treatments, he was able to get the proper texts from the library, make his notes, and then produce two five-page assignments which he excitedly handed in. He was overjoyed to receive an eighty on each. He has shown marked improvement in comprehension, reading, writing, and mechanical ability. He has been asked to return for monthly check-up visits. There is also room for further improvement. Just prior to this book going to press, Louis called and told the authors he had received a 2.97 score for his semester. This mark is based on the 4.0 formula.

CASE #6:   Kara L.   Age 10   Female

	At Exam	2nd Visit	3rd Visit
Dominance	Right	Right	Right
Gait	Unilateral	Unilateral	Unilateral
Shoe tying	Good	Good	Good
Crawling	Good	Good	Good
Calisthenics	Fair	Fair	Improved*
Directional instruction	Normal	Normal	Normal
Muscle tone	Good	Good	Good
Mechanical ability	Poor	Good*	Good
Colors	Normal	Normal	Normal
Comprehension	Fair	Fair	Good*
Emotions	Fair	Fair	Improved*
Hyperkinesis	Good	Good	Good
Vowel pronunciation	Ragged	Good*	Good
Reading, free	Good	Good	Good
Reading, held	Good	Good	Good
Reading, legs crossed	Good	Good	Good
Writing	Good	Good	Good
Arithmetic	Good	Good	Good
Cloacal reflexes	Six	Four*	Clear**
Cranial faults	Four	Two*	Clear**
Ocular lock	SE & W	Clear**	Clear**

Notes on Case #6, Kara L.: Kara was a very-well-organized ten-year-old girl. She spoke politely and with good diction except for vowel pronunciation.

Her emotional stability was only fair and her athletic prowess ragged. She had a full quota of cranial faults and cloacal reflex abnormalities and two sets of orbital muscle weaknesses. In five visits, Kara was discharged as clear with marked improvement in comprehension, reading, vowel pronunciation, mechanical ability, and a newfound appreciation of humor. It was very interesting to follow this case. Kara attended summer camp, and the new receptivity resulted in more exposure to and greater skill in the various programs made available by a camp experience. She had promised to read for one hour each day while at camp. As in most cases like this, the fact that the child started treatment with a reasonably good score resulted in complete clearance by summer's end. It was a plus for her when it was discovered she was counseling other children in not fearing certain situations instead of experiencing her usual great need for it herself. It has been planned to give Kara some supportive treatment over the next couple of months to smooth off some of the rough edges.

Case #7:   L. S.   Chiropractic physician   43 years of age
He is dyslexic and has been in practice fifteen years. He got through school with a tape recorder and help from his girl friend, who is now his wife. After one treatment, he read a book in four days and then three books in three days. For the first time in his life, he was able to complete a book at all. A follow-up examination/treatment was arranged for three weeks later.

Case #8:   J. S.   Daughter of doctor above
Youngest of five children; others seemed all right and were not examined because they lived in a different state. She was very shy, basically introverted, and read with difficulty, needing a line guide or pointing with a finger. She exhibited emotional problems. After five treatments, she returned home with her father continuing the care; she was in the spring term at the time. In the fall term, after Thanksgiving, she was in two special classes, the rest regular classes. She earned a straight-A average and became the extrovert of the family. She volunteers for everything in school, and her teachers cannot get over the dramatic emotional and scholastic changes in her.

Case #9:   Mike   High school student   17 years of age
Mike tested at grade nine level in the eleventh grade. He needed constant help with homework and assignments. Treatment was commenced one week after school started. Within another week, he was able to complete all assignments without help. Five weeks later, he was retested and found to be at eleventh-grade level. The only concession was to allow a little extra

time for the testing. Mike was shy and withdrawn but is now very involved
in all of his senior-class activities. He had a total of five treatments.

Case #10:   Mathew   Eleven years of age

Mathew is dyslexic and has poor motor coordination and allergies. His
parents would take him to the park on weekends to use the batting cage
and other equipment in the playground in an attempt to improve his motor
skills. After two treatments, he was taken back to the park and was able
to hit thirteen out of twenty balls pitched, where, prior to that, he was lucky
to hit even one. Also, he was able to play miniature golf and get the ball
through mazes and into the holes. Allergies had to be programmed out
because these would create emotional and dyslexic problems on their own.
He has been seen once a month and has remained clear. His schoolwork
has gone from poor to fair to good in all subjects. School and family are
very happy with the result.

Case #11:   Stephan   Eleven years of age

This boy could not tie his shoelaces, was shy but very friendly. He needed
constant help in everything and was in all special classes. Stephan was clear
after eight treatments and has needed no further intervention since in his
monthly visits. He is in all regular classes now, a year and a half later.

Case #12:   V. F.   College student   Nineteen years of age

This boy was struggling to stay in school. He was a football hero. The coach
at first wanted him to be wide receiver because of his speed and put him
on the right side of the line. He would run out, cut left, but could not catch
the ball. If he had been on the left side of the line, he could have caught
over his right shoulder, but the coach made him a running back, would
give him the ball, and he would run with it. He had been relying on tape
recorders and his girl friend to manage his assignments in school. When
questioned as to why he had dropped two English courses, he replied, "Dad,
I can't read." One treatment corrected the problem; he was only learning
disabled, not dyslexic.

Case #13:   R. N.   Female   Twenty-five years of age

This patient is recently married and is working. Her complaints were varied,
mostly dealing with poor digestion and headaches. Examination revealed
the dyslexic components. When questioned, she said she could not read well,
reversed words and letters, and could not spell or do math. She thought
she was just dumb. While she was growing up, everyone told her that she

was dumb, clumsy, didn't have any sense, didn't try hard enough. She accepted this as fact. Three treatments were needed to clear her, at which point she got a new job. She's doing quite well at present.

Case #14:   Michael   Male   Seven years of age
Michael was seven and could not tie shoelaces or button coats properly. He was not being transferred to a special school for problem children. He was well behaved. Teachers, however, said he would not pay attention and did not try to learn anything. His mother claimed differently. The boy was allergic and had asthma. He required eight treatments, and a complete altering of his diet was arranged for. At present he is in regular school and doing adequate work without any extra help.

Case #15:   John   Chiropractic physician's son   Six years of age
John was having problems keeping up with his class although he was getting intensive help at home and special tutoring in the summer. His father was concerned because the school wanted the term repeated. He was treated three times with followup by his father. Before Thanksgiving recess, John was commended by the teacher for the marvelous change that had come over him—as he was second in his class at that time.

7

Examination Factors

Before entering upon the following coverage, it should be stated that the professional appearance of this material is included in order to exhibit the extent to which the kinesiologist must go to determine the basic reasons for the myriad conditions found in the learning disabled. The authors do not wish to discourse at a level over the reader's head, nor do they want this book to be so weighty that confusion could occur. Rather, they feel the need to display the parameters that must be reached in order to accomplish what is required.

THE STRUCTURAL, PHYSIOLOGICAL, AND NEUROLOGIC FACTORS

Once the principles and philosophy of applied kinesiology are understood, the absolute simplicity of the kinesiological survey, examination, and treatment is what makes the procedure so valuable. Kinesiological procedures—which are based in chiropractic, acupuncture (meridian therapy), nutrition, neurology, psychology, orthopedics, reflex therapies, et cetera—are always logical in the sense that the body's functions are always logical, even if we don't yet understand all the logic. They are demonstrable for all to see; they are repeatable by those skilled in the procedures. They are predictable if what is done is neurologically, physiologically, and anatomically correct. A specific result is expected if the body language is followed in examination and treatment; they are reversible. In almost all procedures, one can completely reverse what has been done, start over, or change direction. The authors are unaware of any other technique, treatment, or procedure that can equal this completeness, uniqueness, and absolute scientific basis.

The triad of health is the most important principle to consider. All areas of dysfunction are investigated, treated, and checked for clearance. Faulty nutrition is rectified. The overriding thought always is that anything can cause anything; so by normalizing as many points of imbalance as are found, the chances of removing the negative aspects of dis-ease are very great.

We are still learning, investigating, expanding, refining, and discovering how the body really works. The stress or emphasis in these endeavors is always on organization of all bodily functions. In the case of learning disabilities, the organization and coordination of the neurologic and physiologic functions of the body and brain, the chemical balance, and the psychologic ramifications are what are necessary to eliminate the condition. These factors will be discussed later.

Instead of attempting to teach people afflicted with disabilities to live with them and cope with them, it might be more practical to investigate the kinesiological approach. The neurologic functions can be normalized and the proprioceptor mechanisms balanced and organized. The dysfunction of the eye muscles can be corrected and the chemical balance of the body and brain controlled. Psychological problems can be neutralized so that the information bombarding the senses is processed properly for interpretation, understanding, and use.

Every procedure in the step-by-step process of examination and treatment is tested; those found wanting are corrected and a positive indicator of those dysfunctions should be cleared at that time. This does not mean, however, in most conditions of dis-ease or disease, that the patient is cured or asymptomatic instantly, although in many cases that is what happens. It does mean that the neurologic, physiologic, and anatomic dysfunctions in the body are reordered, recoordinated and reestablished. If tissue healing is a necessary part of the recovery, the body is now responding and the cause is being or has been found. In short order, the patient will be well with little or no residual effects of the debility suffered.

If the condition has been neglected and/or not properly treated for a lengthy hiatus of time, there may be structural or tissue changes of a permanent nature that could set limitations on rehabilitation even if the original cause has been removed.

BODY ORGANIZATION

In order to understand body organization, it would be helpful to understand body disorganization, for this is where one starts to organize or reorganize the body in its homogenous functions.

Dr. David Walther, in his excellent book, *Applied Kinesiology*, volume I, describes two types of disorganization, one termed predictable and the other unpredictable. Over the years, many types of disorganization within the body have been found to be predictable in nature. Certain conditions follow specific patterns, and, therefore, diagnoses may be made readily. These patterns are well known in physiology and neurology, while others are patterns developed in chiropractic, osteopathic, naturopathic, and kinesiologic disciplines. The latter are not prominent in the literature but are certainly equally valid. If the physician is familiar with the aberrant patterns, these malfunctions can be located easily and diagnosed and corrected in most cases.

The body communicates with itself through many signaling mechanisms, such as the nervous system; chemical agents such as enzymes, hormones, et cetera; and the meridian energy system (developed primarily in the Orient).

Although there still are unpredictable disorganization factors which do not follow any known pattern, much of what was considered unpredictable in the past has become predictable through recent research. Most of this new knowledge is found outside the realms of established disciplines, however.

In discovering neurologic switching, adaptive mechanisms, backup systems, and, more recently, backup to the backup systems, the undetected emotional factors, the hidden allergenics and so forth, the extra ingredients necessary to understand these unpredictable disorganizations are now understood and the unpredictable becomes predictable.

One of the major factors found by Goodheart[23] was the phenomenon of switching in the body. This results in confused signaling in the body and messages to the brain, particularly when sending right side impulses to the left brain and left side impulses to the right brain. (We all learned in school somewhere that the left brain controls the right side and the right brain controls the left side of the body). This is still a valid assumption.

The messages thus scrambled or misdirected create what seems to be unpredictable disorganization; the central nervous system is confused, and often symptoms show up on the wrong side of the body or information is misinterpreted.

The twenty-seventh and last point on the kidney acupuncture meridian is located at the juncture of the sternum, first rib, and clavicle on each side. K27 has been called the switchboard between the two sides of the body.[5] It is known as the home of associated points.

Digital stimulation of each side of K27, in conjunction with the umbilicus usually results in removal of the cross patterning or switching. The application should be for about twenty seconds on each side.

The disorganization taking place as a result of switching can be resolved by treatment of K27 as above. This will avoid one of our chief concerns, that of action and thought reversals found in persons with learning disabilities. They tend to do things backward, may have a problem with mathematics, and can get lost very easily, trying to get from one location to another.

An important guide to neurologic integrity is the positive or negative switching found in examination. It pays dividends for the doctor to check K27 on several occasions during the course of treatment so he may keep abreast of changes in the patient's progress. It is always possible to find the patient has switched from one visit to the next.

Goodheart found three main switching mechanisms in the body. They will be referred to as primary. The first is the acupuncture or meridian point found at the upper end of the kidney meridian known as K27. Goodheart describes K27 as the switchboard between the two sides of the body. Occasionally there is another factor associated with K27, located at the transverse process of the eleventh thoracic

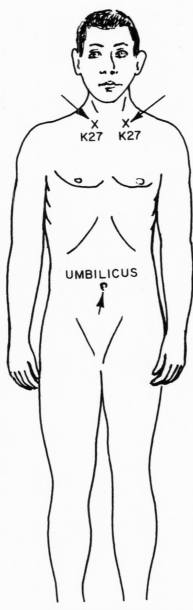

X   X
K27   K27

UMBILICUS

K27 kidney meridian

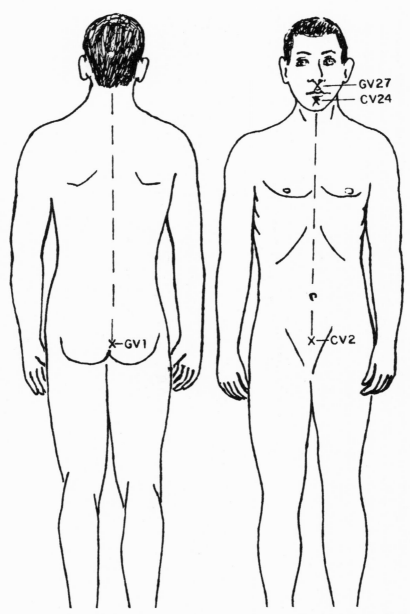

GV27
CV24

X-GV1

X-CV2

Governing vessel meridian   Conception vessel meridian

vertebra bilaterally and is referred to as auxiliary K27.[14] Corrections for these points are accomplished in association with umbilical stimulation (the Oriental center of energy).*

Another switching mechanism also has its origin in the acupuncture meridian circuits. It is designated as the governing vessel. This energy line is located on the posterior of the body. It extends from the tip of the coccyx, upward through the midline on the spine, over the head, and terminates in the gum line under the upper lip. These points are designated as GV1 and GV27, respectively.

The third switching mechanism is found on the energy meridian and is known as the conception vessel. This line is located on the anterior. It extends from the perineum up the midline to the center of the lower lip. The points active in this type of switching are designated as CV2 and CV24, respectively. CV2 is found on the upper border of the symphysis pubis. The associated point for the governing vessel is B16, located between the sixth and seventh thoracic vertebrae. Many times a subluxation is found at this point and must be adjusted in order to clear the vertebral level and switching mechanism.

A lesser-known posterior switching mechanism is also of great importance when considering neural organization. This is located by therapy localizing the tip of the coccyx and the umbilicus. There is an auxiliary point to this mechanism located between the fifth and sixth thoracic vertebrae. As with the auxiliary K27 at the eleventh thoracic vertebra, if a deficiency is found, a regular manipulative adjustment needs to be administered at that level in order to clear the switching mechanism.

While on the subject of body organization, it might be well to consider the fact that athletic agility and endurance depend greatly upon the integrity of the neural organization and, therefore, coordination. An example which comes to mind is that of a runner who, prior to kinesiological treatment, had tried for seven years to better his timing. More will be found on this case in the addendum at the end of the book. The statistics on this case are not a matter of learning disability, but they do contribute to the overall consideration of the importance of balancing the health triad.

*The K27 switching mechanism is also known as the anterior switching mechanism.

Another mechanism which can cause a neural switching problem is that of ocular lock. Simply stated, it is the neural phenomenon associated with the inability of a patient to look in certain directions without causing neural deficit in the body function. This occurs when the muscles of the eyes become strained when using them to look in one or more directions due to the lack of balance in their tension. This is almost always associated with the K27 switching mechanism and was thought by most kinesiologists to be the primary dysfunction in dyslexia and other learning disabilities tied in with reading difficulties.

Patients with the problem are rendered unable to read for any length of time, resulting in poor comprehension, and it requires going back repeatedly on words missed. One finds difficulty in following lines of type without some kind of guide. One oddity about this kind of switching is that although the person finds it very difficult to read from left to right, there is no difficulty in reading from right to left as in Hebrew or Arabic.

The test for ocular lock is to have the patient look in all directions—up, down, right, and left—as well as all the oblique angles. As in all therapy localization, if the test is positive, the body cannot maintain neurologic integrity, and any strong indicator muscle will weaken. Another method of evaluation for ocular lock was developed by Kirshner. While maintaining stress on a strong indicator muscle, he would have the patient follow the examiner's finger with his eyes, completely around in both clockwise and counterclockwise circles. If there is a problem, the indicator muscle will weaken in one or the other of these directions.

By stimulating K27 and the umbilicus, this positive test usually is neutralized, and the eyes will return to normal function, at least for a while. Because of the temporary nature of this correction, in many cases further investigation related this dysfunction to primary respiratory faults of the cranial bones, and unless these also are corrected, the condition returns. This type of switching is most common, and at one time or another, the majority of people will experience it. Because the body is self-healing in most aspects, everyday activity will free the lock and normalcy will return. That is, until stress, fatigue, overindulgence, or whatever environmental or habitual conditions which brought on the dysfunction in the first place can recreate the condition. Specific professional help is needed for a more permanent cure.

According to Goodheart, Walther, et al., there are many factors influencing the switching mechanisms, which then lead to the disorganization of the nervous system and conditions such as dyslexia and other learning disabilities.

CRANIAL PRIMARY RESPIRATORY DYSFUNCTION

An area of major deficit in the healing arts in medical, osteopathic, and certain chiropractic circles is the cranial respiratory motion. Unfortunately, the standard texts say that the cranial bones do not move, and most practitioners look no further. They have accepted with blind faith that this is so and therefore inhibit a major area of investigation into the cause and treatment of many conditions. Dysfunction of the respiratory movement of the cranial bones is involved in most of man's problems to one extent or another. Cranial respiratory function can influence the body in many ways and create, among other things, the condition known as switching. Normal cranial nerve activity appears to be specifically dependent on normal cranial respiratory movement. The considerable amount of sensory input from vision, hearing, taste, smell, feeling, balance, and so forth in this area can easily be confused if the physiological functions of the cranial bones are in fault—the switching phenomena. It is easy to see that if the eyes are not functioning well together with the ears, for example, a strain on the nervous system in its attempt to orient the body to its environment may arise. Bilateral activity, such as the basic gait reflexes, requires bilateral communication in the brain and nervous system. This bilateral activity cannot be developed efficiently if the sensory input is confused, misunderstood, or otherwise dysponetic in nature.[23] It therefore seems reasonable that if the physiologic function of the cranial bones is at fault in any of their many motions (see *cranial function*), neurologic confusion can follow.

Other mechanisms involved in neural disorganization and confusion (switching) are pelvic dysfunctions, including the common sacroiliac and lumbosacral distortions (interfering with proper proprioceptive signaling and gait mechanisms, which are part of our reflex system). Also there are foot dysfunctions (causing many kinds of scrambled messages to the central nervous system) and ionization (proper electrical balance of tissues, organs, and so forth). These factors have not been found to have relation to the basic problem dealt with in this writing up to now but may need to be considered in specific resistant cases.

ORGANIZATIONAL DEVELOPMENT

Normal neural cross-patterning develops during the crawling and then walking stages of early youth. In a properly coordinated, neurologically balanced individual, normal left arm-right leg and right arm-left leg function should be present when an individual walks or crawls. Because this neural organization is basic to the central nervous system function, any deviation from this is cause to suspect a problem. Although this basic pattern of movement, which helps to organize the central nervous system, should be and almost always is developed in very early youth, it can be learned at any age to either organize or, in the case of severe damage, reorganize the central nervous system.

It is important to note here that most learning disabled and dyslexics had, at best, limited crawling experience as young children. The authors feel this is related to dysfunctions of the cloacal centering and righting system. Included here are the labyrinthine and visual righting reflex systems. This dysfunction can be either inborn or acquired due to accident or birth trauma.

CLOACAL SYNCHRONIZATION

Cloacal synchronization is a system of evaluating the cloacal reflexes. Although they are primary sexual centering reflexes in the animal kingdom, they are considered primitive or innate (inborn) centering reflexes in man. The points are located in the anterior and posterior surfaces of the pelvic region. Their activity appears to correlate with the visual righting and labyrinthine reflexes and the tonic neck receptors. In a full evaluation of this system, therefore, we join them in testing and correction when therapy localizing. All of these reflexes are involved with the centering of the body and/or its orientation in space.

The cloacal reflexes center the pelvis. The visual righting and labyrinthine righting reflexes center the head. The tonic neck receptors center the head and neck. Together, they center the head to the body and/or the pelvis to the head. It is clear why this mechanism is so all-important in neural organization and disorganization.

These reflexes also can be evaluated by testing groups of muscles simultaneously. There are eight such sets that may be tested in checking these reflexes. This area of work will not be discussed in this volume.

There is an unusual type of switching found in the cloacal synchronization which involves what is termed the cross K27 factor. This is localized or tested in the reverse manner of normal K27 evaluation. The hands are crossed over each other, care being taken that they do not touch each other. The tips of the fingers of the left hand contact the right side of K27 and the right fingers on the left side, simultaneously. This cross-pattern is associated with a homolateral crawl or gait pattern. This unnatural pattern will be seen in schizophrenics and other individuals with heightened sensory disturbances.[23]

George Goodheart is owed a great debt for his development of the cloacal and labyrinthine reflex system.[9] There seems to be a strong connection with the centering of body balance and awareness.

The posterior cloacal reflex points are located just above the apex of the sacrum on each side (see page 55). They are therapy localized in conjunction with the labyrinthine reflexes, which are found medial to the mastoid process on each side. The therapy localization is done singly and in tandem, with eyes open as well as closed. Cranial correction is made wherever positive findings are met. On rare occasions, the doctor will find that clearance of a positive reflex does not prevail. In this instance, checking both right or both left reflex points simultaneously may bring about synchronization.

There is an apparent signaling that takes place by the altered reflex which throws off the balance of the body in all areas of mechanical and/or chemical integrity. The semicircular canals of the ears are involved with equilibrium and, as such, are responsible for keeping the body in close harmony with the force of gravity.

The anterior cloacal reflex points are located on either side of the pubis on the exterior surfaces of the superior rami (see page 56). The treatment is accomplished here as well as the therapy localization. These points are checked in conjunction with the visual righting (ocular) reflexes which are located medial to the supraorbital notch on the supraorbital margin.

The therapy localization is done singly and in tandem with eyes open as well as closed. Occasionally a homolateral checking, that is, both reflexes on the right or both on the left, must be done, and on a few occasions the authors have found it necessary to check posterior and anterior points simultaneously.

It is recognized that the visual righting reflex should be done with eyes open only, according to presently available texts,[7] but the authors have found that the closed-eye test was applicable, especially where a person has had a head injury and had the eyes closed at that moment.

In the case of a learning disability, positive findings are quite common in most instances in the cloacal and visual righting reflexes, and the correction results in dramatic clearance almost immediately.

THE IMPORTANCE OF THE BODY LANGUAGE OF SWITCHING

As we have seen, there are many causes of switching. It is a neural phenomenon which involves confusion in an otherwise ordered nervous system and can lead to or cause many problems in the body function, i.e., the chronic low back pain or other spinal problems to which a vast number of our population are prone, the chronic headaches, as well as digestive, bowel, and glandular abnormalities, and almost all other infirmities of mankind. This is not to say that this is the only cause, but in the authors' experience, switching plays a major role in the everyday health care rendered in the office.

The reader should consider this in the context of the foregoing— the reversal of action or thought is probably the most often recognized sign of the disorganized nervous system. The patient does exactly

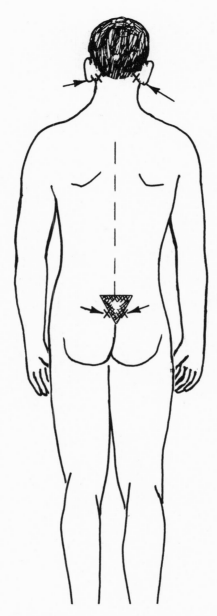

Posterior cloacal and labyrinthine reflexes

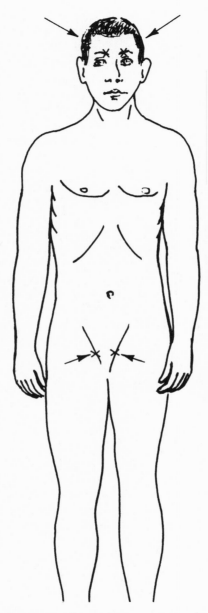

Anterior cloacal and ocular righting reflexes

opposite of what is directed or requested. "Lie on your back" becomes face down. "Turn right" results in going left. "Look down" becomes up. Reversals are common in the transportation of letters in typing, numbers in mathematics, and making statements or using words opposite to what is meant.[23] Does this sound familiar?

Switching often is manifest in poor coordination of the musculoskeletal system. Children and/or adults may have poor coordination in catching, throwing, or hitting a ball. Both men and women will evidence unaccountable bruises on their legs and arms from continually bumping into furniture, doorjambs, or even the doors themselves. Dropping or spilling things constantly is another indication. A severely switched child generally is the "klutz" of the playground, the last to be chosen in a game, the one who can't seem to get out of his own way. Many times when dominance has not been established, the child will tend to throw or catch a ball with either hand. He is neither a "rightie" nor a "leftie," although many tend to be left-handed in the use of pen or pencil.

The switched patient is usually awkward, while the organized patient has a rhythm to his movements while walking or running. Usually, the doctor does not have the opportunity to observe the patient during outdoor activities, so this all-important body language is not readily available for evaluation. These factors should be discussed, therefore, with the patient or the patient's parent. If there is any lack of balance or rhythm in rapid movement, switching should be suspected. If the arms and/or legs flail awkwardly, there may be a problem.

Another condition associated with switching is that of stuttering, and although the child or adult learns to overcome this affliction, the neurologic disorganization which caused it in the first place may remain, only to promote other health problems.[23] Many times the condition is corrected with ease by what seems to be simple unswitching technique to reorganize the nervous system. A qualified kinesiologist can make the evaluation necessary to determine the failure of neurologic organizational development.

RIGHT AND LEFT DOMINANCE

One-sided dominance usually is associated with neural integrity.

The dominance should be one-sided. That is, if the person is right-handed, he should be right-eyed, right-eared, and right-footed as well. Deviation of any part of this conformity to organization makes an individual a likely candidate for switching. Because kinesiology is very specific in almost all of its examination and treatment procedures, treatment can be directed to any one of the many conditions associated with switching.[23]

Ideally, the eyes should function together efficiently so that no matter in what direction or how far in that direction the eyes are moved, no neural deficit occurs when the eyes continue to function together. When they do not, ocular lock is the usual result. A well-developed organization requires a dominant eye function. If there is poor organizational development of dominancy or ocular lock, the dominancy will shift from eye to eye so that they tend never to center upon an object but rather constantly shift their gaze. This body language will give the first indication of switching to an experienced kinesiologist.[23]

A poor reader often is found to have abnormal neural organization. A person with a learning disability related to reading always has poor neural organization. The eyes do not coordinate in balanced movement; the eye muscles do not allow both eyes to function properly together. Therefore, the individual finds it difficult, if not impossible, to follow the lines down a page. If nothing else, the difficulty in following the written or printed word from line to line results in eye fatigue, distraction, and poor sensory input. Dyslexia is a classic example of this type of switching in which we see reversals of words, letters and symbols, and mirror-image reading or writing.

When an individual sees the word "saw" and reads it as "was," one can readily see that this can lead to much confusion on the part of a new reader trying to make some sense out of what he is trying to learn to read. Often, all that is necessary to correct a simple learning disability (not dyslexia) is a reorganization or first-time organization of the nervous system through techniques available in applied kinesiology.[23]

If an individual tends to go to sleep or gets very tired or eye-weary as soon as he starts to read, it is fairly certain that this is another example of neural disorganization manifesting itself with the use of the eyes. The neurologic insult or neural deficit created by the attempt to use the eyes in a coordinated manner, as in reading, can be dramatically and instantly demonstrated by applying the simple intact muscle test used in kinesiological examination. It is thought that the muscle weakening resulting in the discoordinated eye muscle function turns off the entire body because all muscles tested will be weak, thus sleepiness develops from attempted reading.[23]

The value of knowing there is a body language of switching other than that of evaluating a particular patient and his problems is that he can understand his own problems better. He can know what aspects of his health economy relate to this dysfunction. If he also understands that there seems to be an inherited tendency for certain kinds of switching, he can relate this information to immediate family and relatives. Heretofore unexplained behavior or overlooked conditions can be more readily recognized and help sought for them. Often, a doctor using kinesiology will hear, "So that's why my child can't read, do math, play ball, et cetera."[23]

Often, an uninitiated new patient will think this different kind of doctor has a crystal ball or uses ESP when he is asked if he is a poor reader, or tires quickly when attempting to concentrate on the printed word, or says or does the opposite from what he means.

Most patients will not discuss these kinds of problems with the doctor, particularly in the beginning. They are embarrassed, feel they are just not as smart as others, or they do not relate this problem to others they might have. Perhaps they are unaware they have a problem because they think this is the way they are and have accepted the fact. In other cases, when they are fully aware of the problem and have even had special educational experiences related to it, they were told nothing else could be done for them; therefore they do not bring up the subject.

The patient being treated by kinesiological methods is quick to realize that the procedure is different from all others he or she has experienced. His many problems have been seen to be thoroughly understood, and a solid rapport is established. Healing is therefore accelerated.

The evidence indicates that the manifestations of the symptoms of switching seem to develop in patterns. If the individual has musculoskeletal disorganization, it is rare he will have a learning, reading, or clear-thinking disorganization. There are some people, however, who are so completely switched or disorganized, there are significant problems in both areas.[23] With the exception of the last statement, this seems to be fortunate in a sense. It is as if the people with learning, reading, or other disabilities have enough against them, trying to cope with life in general, without structural aches and pains to complicate matters even more. Those with musculoskeletal problems, on the other hand, have enough trouble getting through life in pain. Unfortunately, because learning disability does not cause pain, they are not likely to seek the doctor who can be of the most help to them. One of the purposes of this book is to explore the values of kinesiology and enlighten the reader with the possibilities.

8

Equilibrium Proprioceptors

Equilibrium proprioception is an essential part of the neural signaling into the central nervous system in relation to organization. It allows the animal (and man) to orient to the environment, that is, the body position and posture in relation to its external location and the body parts to the body parts. Overall, the equilibrium proprioception mechanism is part of the defense or reflex system, necessary for survival of the species.

A brief discussion follows as to the various reflex systems and how they relate to the overall or total problem of dyslexia and learning disabilities.

It is important to restate the purpose of some of the technical data presented up to now and what will follow. This material is intended for the layman as well as the professional. So that these segments of the population know that this new and unique approach is different, is based on sound neurologic, physiologic, and anatomic processes and *does* work, the technical information is presented on the various mechanisms involved.

Neural organization is the basis and the key to the treatment of and a relief from dyslexia and other learning disabilities. When we consider the gait problem a dyslexic has (even when it seems to be overcome), the equilibrium problems, and the general disorganization of the interpretive neural mechanism, it is easier to understand the absolute necessity for total organization of the body and its functions.

LABYRINTHINE RIGHTING REFLEXES

The labyrinthine righting reflexes are related to the inner ear. These reflexes are stimulated or activated by the varied head positions. They then reflexly cause the cervical musculature to react and orient the head to gravity. A cat or other animal held upside down by its feet will turn its head into proper relationship with gravity, even if the eyes (visual righting reflex) are blindfolded, thus demonstrating this reflex action.[23]

BODY ON HEAD REFLEX

Asymmetrical pressure on the surface of the body causes the trunk and limb muscles to right the body and orient it to the head, whether supine, prone, or side-lying. Sometimes the skin reflexes have to be corrected or reset due to trauma.[23]

NECK RIGHTING REFLEXES

The joint receptors of the cervical spine, particularly the first, second, and third vertebrae, are activated or stimulated when a side-lying animal whose head is oriented with gravity will orient its body to its head.[23] The proprioceptors in the neck play an important role in maintaining orientation in space and the ability to function in a normal manner.[29] Anesthetic block to the dorsal roots of C1 through 3 causes severe defects in balance, orientation, and motor coordination. The effects are on motor activity of the total body rather than being localized to a particular structure or area.[29] Manipulative adjustments are needed many times in this area, as subluxations or other dysfunctions of the upper cervical or occipital region can influence muscular function throughout the body.[23]

VISUAL RIGHTING REFLEXES

Most of us have experienced the disorientation in equilibrium when we went to the fun house at an amusement park where the room was set at an angle to gravity. The visual confusion disoriented the body balance and coordination. It sent information into our central nervous system that did not jibe with our other reflex organization, therefore, the confusion. If an animal is surgically labyrinthectomized and held upside down as previously described, it will still orient its head to gravity if the visual mechanism is intact. If blindfolded, it will no longer have the instinct to right the head.[23]

We can now begin to see that the righting and equilibrium mechanisms have considerable input for proper function and organization of the central nervous system. It is further evident when we consider the work of Twitchell, who states that new reactions are not added to higher levels of the nervous system but the primitive reactions become modified and elaborated as the stimulus for their response becomes more discriminating, that is, information added to the primitive reflexes in the normal individual.[31]

CLOACAL REFLEX SYSTEM

Although the cloacal reflex system is not described in standard physiology texts, there is evidence of its existence and function in the human. Its function in lower animals is the centering of the male to the female in genital contact, and new evidence indicates that this function extends to man although it is not as necessary to sexual activity.

The cloacal reflex system has been referred to as primitive. Basically this means it is an inborn or innate system needing no training or other learning technique. In man, the evidence is that this system functions as a centering device for the pelvis in all body positions. This reflex system works automatically from birth and integrates and works in conjunction with the labyrinthine, head and neck, visual righting, and other reflexes. This combination is not only responsible for the centering of the body and its orientation in space and environment, it also is the basis or underlying mechanism for the gait reflex patterns. These we know are the essentials in the normal neural organization of the body.

Another way of looking at this reflex system is that not only does it have its own innate function of centering the body and its parts, it also centers the head (labyrinthine and visual righting reflex) and the pelvis (anterior and posterior cloacal reflex system). In its correlated function, it centers the head to the pelvis, and the pelvis to the head. This system can be considered the raw computer chips upon which the various gait mechanisms of the body (walking, running, turning, sidestepping, and so forth) are ultimately etched. This gait etching or ingraining starts with crawling as a child, later toddling, and finally walking. Eventually, all of the learned body movements of running, dancing, ball playing, and jumping, to name a few, are part of the millions of gait possibilities dependent upon integration of an intact, functioning cloacal, labyrinthine visual righting reflex system.

Once this is understood, it becomes obvious how this reflex system is related to an organized, integrated neural integrity that can process information fed into it and then use it properly.

Some chiropractic techniques used for spinal balancing, such as Spinal Touch, Logan Basic, and other reflex-type methods, are among those which apparently deal with the cloacal reflex system. Applied kinesiology has devised several methods to evaluate the integration of the cloacal, labyrinthine, neck receptor, and visual righting reflexes with other aspects of the body. Because of the excellent clinical response to improved body organization, a very workable hypothesis has been developed.[23]

The testing areas for the posterior cloacal reflex system for pelvic centering are located on the fourth and fifth tubercles of the sacrum and the lateral margins of the coccyx. The locations for the anterior cloacal reflex system for pelvic centering are on the anterior external surface of the superior rami of the pubic bones along the superior border of the obturator foramina. Both of these were located by Beardall and are shown on pages 55 and 56 respectively, in chapter 7.

These test areas also can be used for treatment by vigorous stimulation. In the article "Dyslexia and Learning Disabilities Cured," Dr. Ferreri states that he has found the tips of the ischia to be equally sensitive in therapy localizing the posterior cloacal centering reflexes. Beardall has devised a series of muscle tests to determine the integrity of the various reflexes and their combinations and coordination. For our purposes in this technique, Ferreri has found the therapy localization of these reflexes to be adequate without the necessity of going through the series of muscle tests.

THE LABYRINTHINE RIGHTING REFLEX

The labyrinthine righting reflexes are responsible for orienting the head to gravity correctly and giving the body a sense of balance and stability. These receptors are located in the inner ear. They consist of the semicircular canals and utricles. Although they work independently of the other righting reflexes (that is, they can be tested independently as previously stated), the most important function is that of coordinating with the other centering and/or righting reflex systems to form an integrated balance and centering mechanism for proper body function.

It is obvious that improper signaling from the labyrinthine receptor system will have a profound effect on the postural musculature and body organization due to disturbance in balance. There is much clinical evidence to support this hypothesis.

As with all functions of this type in the body organization, there is a direct cranial primary respiratory system involvement, particularly taking into consideration that the entire hearing and labyrinthine mechanism is located in or on the temporal bone. Barring any specific pathology to this mechanism, the cranial respiratory motion is always involved.[24]

The therapy localization area and treatment contact point for the labyrinthine reflex system (see page 66) is found in the digastric fossa of the temporal bone. There are actually three points located vertically in this fossa, corresponding to slightly different balance functions, and it is best to therapy localize all of them at once. If this reflex is particularly active, the area will be quite painful to the touch, due to the irritated fibers of attachment for the digastric, splenius capitus, and longus capitus muscles.

THE VISUAL RIGHTING REFLEX

The eyes provide a tremendous amount of information for our computer banks. One of the very important factors of the eyes in the optimum function of the organization of the body and its orientation in space and environment is the visual righting reflex. Although a blind person can function adequately in most activities (and some

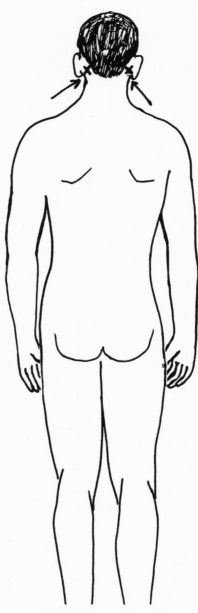

Labyrinthine reflex system

much better than others due to better adaptation), there is obvious disorganization of the body modules, that is, the body posture of head on neck, neck on trunk, trunk on pelvis, et cetera[16] (see page 68).

Most, if not all, of the literature involving the visual righting reflex operates only with the eyes open. Further investigation has indicated that there is a very definite function of this reflex system still active and important in the organization of the gait mechanisms, posture, and the reactive muscle systems, with the eyes closed. The above, therefore, has been renamed or additionally named the ocular righting reflex system.[24] This mechanism will be discussed at greater length in other writings soon to be published. Steve DeVore, in his "Neuropsychology of Achievement," has stated that some of the latest research has indicated that the eye has many nonvisual functions, and many of these have to do with awareness, investigation, coordination, and so forth.

It is important to note that all the above reflex systems are tested separately and together in both homolateral and contralateral positions, with the eyes open in all phases and with the eyes closed in all phases. Occasionally this is done in the dark, occasionally sitting or standing, and sometimes including eye options as part of the examination and treatment procedure. This would depend upon the patient's particular idiosyncrasies. In this way, we are dealing with the total integration of the nervous system in its relation to these orientation and coordination reflex systems and their relation to switching and disorganization of the central nervous system.

The body has balance and awareness mechanisms active in the light and others or extensions of these systems in the dark. *This is with the eyes open as well as closed.* All this must be taken into consideration when one is dealing with organization and coordination of the nervous system. This is more particularly true when we are handling learning disabilities and dyslexia, which are manifestations of profound disorganization and discoordination of the nervous system.

CORRECTION

There are three methods of correction or treatment for synchronizing the cloacal, labyrinthine, and ocular reflex systems. The

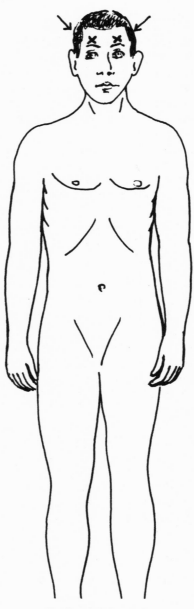

Ocular righting reflex

methods are described by Goodheart. One is simply a moist hand contact held until the area pulsates or until the combined areas pulsate in unison. Another is to gently manipulate the associated structures into their normal physiological respiratory motion as related to the cranial-sacral primary respiratory system. A third method is to stimulate the reflex points vigorously.

The corrections are always made as the faults are found. If they are found to be contralateral anterior cloacal and ocular, the correction is made in that phase. Goodheart advises to "fix it the way you find it."

9

The Cranial Involvements Found in Dyslexia and Learning Disabilities

The primary respiratory motion, as mentioned earlier, is a physiological function that is the basis of maintaining life in the body. It is responsible for all of the vital functions in one way or another. Yet, there is controversy in and among the healing professions even as to its very existence, let alone how it influences the various life forces.

Everything moves when we breathe, from the arches in our feet to the top of our skull. The first thing we do to allow ourselves to function outside the uterus is to take our first breath. If we continue to breathe, we live; if we don't, we die. This seemingly simplistic and rather obvious statement has far-reaching and very vital applications for all living creatures. Respiration is not the mere exchange of gases, as most assume if and when they think of the breathing process at all. Respiration is a vital force that drives the machinery of life.

The diaphragm is our most important muscle, not the heart, as most everyone would agree. The large bellows that divides the body in half acts as a reciprocal action pump that not only creates a suction or vacuum to suck air into the lungs but then causes a compression to expel the air from the lungs. This is the respiratory function everyone knows of.

There is an equally vital function of the diaphragm that is much less recognized. The movements of the diaphragm create a major hydraulic drive mechanism, for one thing, to assist the heart in pumping the blood throughout the body. The heart pumps the blood down through the aorta and the femoral arteries to the lower body and extremities. It then creates a suction to help lift the blood back up the body, along with other muscle activity to return it to the heart. It also helps to push the blood up to the head and pull it back down again. So far, these are simple to understand and are obvious functions of the diaphragm. A more sophisticated action is the effect the diaphragm itself has on the lymphatic system. The volume of blood pumped to the extremities cannot circulate back through the venous system immediately. Because of the necessity of purifying it, the design was to not totally return directly to the heart for recirculating. A major portion of the fluid of the blood is returned to the circulation through the lymph system. It is first processed or purified through a series of lymph glands which are miniature "sewage disposal plants" or filters. This is similar to a filter on a pool; to keep it operating, it must be periodically back-flushed. The mechanical hydraulic pressure causes a constant reverse flow for the lymph glands, thereby maintaining their function. In spite of this constant back-flush, occasionally they get plugged up and problems arise.

An even more sophisticated, intricate, and vital function derives from a series of ligamentous attachments which connect to the vertebrae, pelvis, and skull. A physiologic motion is thereby maintained. This is important in allowing for certain reflex actions, neural functions for proprioception and balance, and a minimal motion of all structures to maintain their integrity and prevent fixation. Life is constant activity and motion; it never stops. If it does, the result is self-evident.

There is a continuity of fascia from the apex of the diaphragm to the base of the skull. This fascial connection extends to the various attachments on the occipital, sphenoid, and temporal bones on their outer surfaces. This facilitates a motion of the skull, coordinated with the respiration process and the movement of the diaphragm. This fascial connection then extends through the foramina found in the base of the skull to wrap around the vessels and nerves and join the dura. Traction on intracranial structures has been observed when the head is put into either flexion or extension.[29]

The connections are part of the mechanism involved in the respiratory motion found in all structures of the body, particularly the skull. We are considering, therefore, a mechanism that not only creates a mechanical impetus to move both gases and fluids around the body but also causes movements such as tugging, twisting, and so forth, that maintain integrity of the tissues. All body tissues must be in a reasonably constant motion. For example, if it becomes necessary to immobilize a limb with a cast or brace, measurable connective tissue degeneration can be determined in just four hours, using electromyography as the measuring device.

The cranial respiratory mechanism and the normal intrinsic pulsations of all organs are responsible for the creation of cerebrospinal fluid. It also controls the circulation of that vital juice of life and the milking of the pituitary gland. It generally maintains the vitality of the central nervous system and its control of life forces.

It is important that the reader understand and know that there is movement of the cranial bones. This movement takes place in a rhythmic manner, and the normal physiologic motion can be interrupted by imbalance, subluxation, or fixation, causing neurologic deficit. This text cannot go into all the possible movements of the cranial bones or a full explanation of the mechanisms involved and their ultimate ramifications. When one considers that there are more than one hundred articulations in the skull, it is easy to see that this great number of surfaces collectively allows for a relatively large range of motion. These individual articulations can have so many interactions, in a structure the size of the skull, that the possibility of subluxation (malalignment), restriction of motion, or flexion of even one bone with its several articulations is highly possible. This alteration, restriction, or change in any way from the normal physiological motion of any one of the cranial bones will alter the physiologic motion and function of all related bones. Since the skull is the repository of the brain, the various cranial motions were designed to help maintain the balance, support, protection, circulation, and stimulation of the brain. Therefore, it will bear repeating that any alteration of the physiologic motions of the cranial bones will have some degree of adverse effect on the functions of the brain.

External and internal factors must be considered when contemplating either the specific or more general restriction or subluxation of cranial motion. External influences are some of the more obvious. Trauma of any kind will impact on the body, causing tension. This usually will register on the highly reactive trapezius muscle. The trapezius has both muscle and fascial attachments to the skull. It also has the pull of other attached muscles and fascia and postural tension. Environmental irritations, such as extremes in temperature, light, or humidity may be considered. Internal influences are mainly from stress on the reciprocal tension membranes of the skull or cord.[30] Also important are nutritional aspects of the diet of the individual and allergies, particularly if relating to the central nervous system. These would cause swelling of the brain, producing stress and tension on the whole cranial mechanism.

The skull is mobile and not a rigid container as once (and still is, in some circles) thought. Therefore, motion is essential to its function. Any strain, restriction, or distortion of motion can be serious. The brain needs more oxygen by weight than any other organ in the body. The respiratory motion of the skull helps in maintaining a higher degree of circulation in that area, thereby assuring the increased oxygen demand of the brain tissue. Given any interference with this function, neurologic deficit or worse can occur.

All organ systems of the body are directly related to one or more of the cranial nerve tracts. Restriction or distortion of the dural membranes can involve one of these tracts or can inflict a variety of neurologic problems because they are firmly attached to all sutures of the cranial cavity.

Another important consideration when dealing with the reciprocal tension membranes and the position and motion of the cranial bones is the basic circulation of the brain and skull. Arterial blood enters the skull unimpeded through arteries which are firm, muscularly walled vessels. The walls of the veins differ in that they are thin and easily compressed. They exit the cranium through holes between the bones that are known as foramina. It is obvious that they are susceptible to soft tissue tension, edema from irritation and subluxation, causing a buildup of pressure within the skull. The headaches and other neurological phenomena are related to this arrangement.[30]

The brain is floating in, cushioned by, partially nourished by, and generally maintained by the cerebrospinal fluid. Any disturbance or change in the physiology of this fluid, either in makeup, density, circulation, or pressure can cause marked alterations in the metabolism of the physiological and psychological centers within the brain. It should be obvious, in view of the cranial function, that any distortion within the skull can and will cause problems, either neurologic, psychologic, physiologic, or any combination thereof.

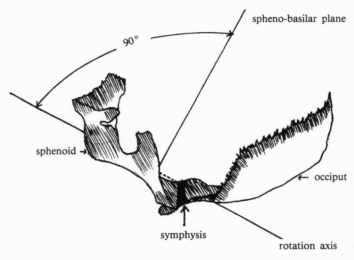

Lateral view of occiput and sphenoid from left side

The primary or basic cranial movement is the spheno-basilar motion. All other cranial motions essentially depend upon this as the impetus for the others. This motion is the flexion and extension movement of the sphenoid and the occiput (see above). The sphenoid is the center bone of the skull and articulates with twelve other cranial bones. It has four motions, all of which go on at the same time. The sphenoid movement is the prime force in all other cranial function. The first of these movements is the rocking or what is otherwise called the flexion and extension, as it articulates with the occiput and forms the spheno-basilar mechanism as noted above.

This motion is the primary pump for the cerebrospinal fluid circulation, the milking of the pituitary gland, and production of the cerebrospinal fluid itself. (There are other functions to consider but that is not the purpose of this text.) A dyslexic will have this motion in fault, usually in the extension phase.

The second motion of the sphenoid is the twisting, torquing, or lateral rocking motion. This also is at fault in the dyslexic, with the bone usually hung up or fixated high on the right, as previously stated. This motion is a very important one in right brain/left brain coordination, gait mechanisms, reciprocal motion of the temporal bone, as well as in polarity. In the reversals of dyslexia, this is the key distortion.

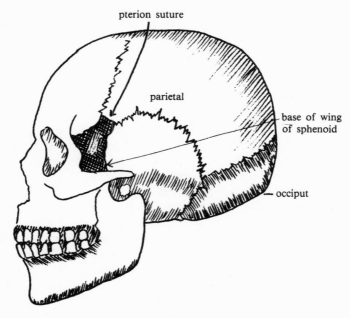

Pterion suture

The sphenoid bone is crucially important in the management of the learning disabled. At times because of the rigors of birth, at times because of acquired injury, at times because of neurological or chemical trauma, this bone becomes slightly displaced and, lacking an opposing force, remains in the unbalanced position. With three exceptions to date, the authors have found this displacement to be only in one direction, that of the lateral surface portion of the greater wing being superior on the right, to that of the left surface. This gives the bone the effect of slanting uphill from left to right. In palpation, the upper ridge, which joins at the frontal and parietal sutures, appears to be more prominent and slightly higher on the right side, while the left shows a palpable depression. Using therapy localization, it is found that contact on these two spots will elicit a weak indicator muscle if the fault is present. The torsion of the sphenoid may be combined with a similar but opposite twisting of the occiput.

The correction is easily accomplished. A light pressure downward is exerted with the heel of the hand on the ridge of the high side. Simultaneously, the left hand assists in a lifting motion on the low side. This should be repeated four or five times, each with an inspirational assist. Also, a headward pressure is exerted on the pterygoid process, back of the last molar, on the inferior side of slant. This must be done with care.

It is at the point of the pterion suture that the tipping of the sphenoid bone may be ascertained. The uppermost border of the bone should mesh smoothly with that of the parietal and be slightly superimposed on it. This is a sliding suture. If a prominent ridge is palpated on one side (usually the right), while a depression is found at the base of the sphenoid wing on the other side, it can be established that the sphenoid is tipped upward on the side showing the ridge and downward on the depressed side.

The third motion of the sphenoid is the lateral spread of the wings. Because of eye muscle attachments to the wings, it can be seen that both the torquing and spreading movements would have bearing on the eye muscle function.

The fourth motion of the sphenoid is one of flexion. This may be involved in dyslexia. All bones flex one way or another, as Dr. H. J. Magoun, in his book, *Osteopathy in the Cranial Field*, states in relation to the cranial bones. Every bone must have sufficient plastic resiliency in itself and enough mobility in its sutures to move through its normal range without strain.[30]

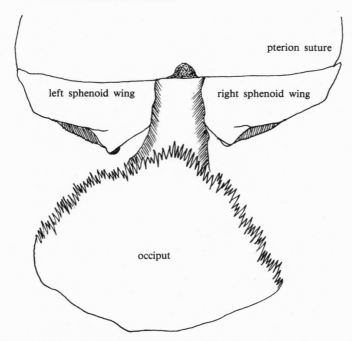

Exaggerated view of torsion and tilt of occiput (low on right) and sphenoid (high on right)

The temporal bones move in reciprocal motion. A fault in the temporal bone movement is part of the dyslexic condition. One or both temporal bones may be at fault, but at least one is necessary in diagnosing dyslexia. We know that a dyslexic suffers a disequilibrium as part of the many problems he must face. The total ear mechanism is located in or on the temporal bone. It is known that a major part of our equilibrium comes from the inner ear structure called the cochlea. The motion of fluid in the cochlea and semicircular canals stimulates cilia, the hairlike projections on the walls of the canals. This constant motion sends a continuous feedback to the brain, giving us balance and/or equilibrium. As was said, the temporal bones move in reciprocal action as they rotate and flare constantly. Any interference with this motion will affect the equilibrium to some degree.

These are the basic cranial faults found in and necessary for the diagnosis of dyslexia. There is a percentage of dyslexics who improve in almost everything, but they tend to retain reversals and there is little change in handwriting. This has been more prevalent in adult female patients. In searching for the reason, we find an emotional "lock" on the reversals, going back to the frustration and embarrassment that this caused them in their childhood and in school. In these cases, other cranial bones come into the picture, e.g., the frontal bone which is generally found to be involved in emotional problems. Occasionally the zygomatics will be found to be at fault. These are the other bones to which the eye muscles are attached. Again it appears that there should be and is a correlation between proper functions of eye, cranial structure, and neurologic control. More discussion will appear in a later chapter on the eye involvement.

Proper cranial function and balance have a direct relation to brain facility. Structure and function are always related. This is dramatically demonstrated in kinesiological treatment. As the cranial corrections are made, the patient many times remarks that he feels different, sees differently, is no longer confused. The nervous system can respond that quickly. One set of parents remarked that they knew they had a different child in the car as they drove home from their first visit.

10

Ocular Lock Phenomenon

A condition named "ocular lock" has been recognized in applied kinesiology for some time. It has had various roots and in the so-called normal person was related to the K27/umbilicus switching mechanism. Most times, it is a temporary condition and simple treatment of the K27 and umbilicus areas instantly clears it. Ocular lock, as previously described, is a neural deficit created by the use of the eyes in certain directions so that muscles weaken, eyes get heavy, motion is hard to follow, and it is difficult to read and coordinate lines of print. Sometimes the ocular lock phenomenon is associated with the sphenoid wing malfunction. This can be therapy localized, treated, and cleared.

Because of the attachments of the eye muscles to the cranial bones, specifically the orbital portions of the sphenoid, frontal, zygomatic, and maxilla, the usual correction of the ocular lock does not follow here. The unswitching done up to now with the correction of the cloacal, ocular, and labyrinthine reflex mechanisms, the all-important K27/umbilicus mechanism, and the cranial bone corrections has integrated and organized the nervous system. The patient now is ready for the final step. The usual ocular lock phenomenon has been eliminated, yet the eyes still react in neural deficit when used in normal fashion. This is because the cranial bones probably have been in subluxation since birth, and the fascia of the eye muscles has become shortened in certain directions. For this reason, the eye muscles cannot function to full potential or with facilitation or defacilitation.

79

(Note: Facilitation is the phenomenon of conservation of energy within the body. When a muscle or group of muscles is put into use, the opposing muscles not being used are turned off or defacilitated. This allows the action to go on unopposed by the muscles not being used.)

Because the muscles of the eyes have been attached to bones that have been subluxated for a long period, they have changed their normal length and therefore can work only with stress and neural deficit. Because these muscles also control the shape of the eyeball, the focus of the eye is sometimes affected. Direct treatment to the eye muscles is necessary in order to help this part of the condition, and this is the ultimate key to the treatment and correction of learning disabilities and dyslexia.

To test for this specific problem, an indicator muscle is chosen as in any therapy localization procedure. The patient is then asked to look in all directions of a circle, without turning the head. When weakness of the indicator muscle is observed or felt, the direction of the eyes is noted. Correction is made into the direction of weakness with a respiratory assist. This is accomplished by having the patient look in the direction of greatest weakness. While maintaining this, but with the eyes closed, the eyeballs are gently stretched in the same direction. This lengthens the attached muscles. This should be repeated in all directions of weakness until the full circle is clear. At this point, the patient should be able to follow the examiner's finger in full circle both clockwise and counterclockwise without any neural deficit being noted. Complete freedom of motion of the eyes without quivering or asymmetrical movement should be the result.

This entire procedure is then repeated, contacting K27. Any corrections necessary are made while maintaining contact. This stage is essential to establish hand/eye coordination, which includes holding a book or pencil in one hand. An interesting test at this point is to have the patient read some printed matter. If the eye muscles were clear with nothing being held, and the patient contacts K27 and then holds the book and attempts to read, a new set of deficiencies may show up. When these are corrected with the K27 contact, the procedure may now be repeated, using a cross-K27 contact. Again, new deficits may show up.

These procedures permit the eyes to function in all the various aspects of normal use without creating neural deficit. These are usually the final steps in neural organization of the learning disabled or dyslexic. Additional techniques will be discussed in a later chapter.

It is interesting to note that in new research being done at Yale University, psychologists Bonnie B. Meskin and Jerome L. Singer noted specific eye movement shifts when patients were asked various questions. Depending upon the type of information asked for, the eyes naturally and subtly shifted in particular directions as though the movement aided the accessibility of the data.

In examining Meskin and Singer, DeVore concluded that the eyes apparently act as a trigger to open up certain types of sensory recall. By consciously and intentionally moving the eyes in a particular direction, you can strengthen and fortify your ability to recall instantly certain types of information. The unimpeded eye motions also aid in the ability to read, learn, and understand.

DeVore discovered that if a person who is right-handed, for example, wishes to activate visual memory, he can do so most effectively when his eyes are in the upper left quadrant. Auditory memory causes the eyes to look laterally left. With emotions and feelings, the eyes are shifted in a lower left position. In body motions, eyes are shifted toward the lower right.

It is even more interesting when it is realized that in most of the eye option failures, the eyes are found up to the left, lateral left, lower left, and lower right.

The eye movements are most essential in body and neural organization and have been referred to as the gateway to the mind. We have learned that the eye, as well as being an organ of vision, has many nonvisual functions, one of which was discussed in the section of ocular righting reflex, giving the body orientation, both with the eyes open and closed.[32]

11

Parental Response before the Fact

LACK OF AWARENESS

Examination of records has revealed that of all parents of learning disabled children, the greatest number are found to be unaware that any real problem exists. They might think the child is a so-called slow learner, an underachiever who needs a lot of prodding with his homework. Or perhaps he is a superactive kid who somehow doesn't seem to carry out requests very readily, neatly, or with good grace. He might be clumsy and not that great with a ball and bat but otherwise doesn't appear to have a problem. He may also be quite active in most sports, socially popular, involved in most things, and just not getting the marks he should be getting. He may be good in some subjects, poor in others, not consistent in any. It is assumed that he just needs to put a little more effort into schoolwork and everything will be fine. "No, he doesn't have a problem; he's just a little slow, or he needs to apply himself a little more, or he doesn't pay attention the way he should. He's preoccupied with other things. He'll be all right." This parent isn't hiding from anything. The fact that there might be something wrong never is considered. Because no one has suggested that the child has a problem, the parents never question him specifically as to why his schoolwork is not up to par. They don't realize that the child is trying so very hard to make it, secretly feels he is just dumb, doesn't understand why he can't read for any length of time. He also knows he doesn't comprehend what he reads, is embarrassed, frustrated, and generally ashamed that he is not living up to expectations.

If a child falls into this general category, the parent should ask specific questions and find out if he is able to read for any length of time (more than twenty minutes), and if he can comprehend the meaning of what has been read after five to ten minutes have elapsed. The results may be surprising!

Occasionally, one of these children is brought in for a checkup or with a digestive complaint or sinusitis. In the course of examination, neural disorganization is found to be a dominant factor. A little judicious questioning and a few additional tests elicit a major switching problem. The child has a comprehension difficulty and avoids ball playing and other similar activities. Another learning disabled has just been found.

One such patient was a boy of eleven whose mother was concerned because her son was spending more time in the nurse's office than he spent in his classroom. His complaint always was the same; he had stomachaches two and three times daily. The mother, when she brought the boy into the office, was asked whether the stomachaches persisted into his home hours, playtime, or mealtime. The answer was no, so it didn't take much imagination to see that he was trying to avoid something at school. Further, it was found that the pains occurred at certain times during the schoolday, indicating that certain subjects were particularly stressful to this boy. The pains were real enough but it almost seemed he could bring them on at will. Actually, it was a simple neurologic phenomenon. It was found that the valve connecting the small intestine to the large intestine or colon would open under stress, causing a sudden accumulation of gas, which, of course, caused severe pain.

The important fact in that case was that not only was the offending valve taken care of, but the learning problems which were quite evident by this time were tackled. The end result was relief from the stomachaches, improved school performance, plus an avid desire to run around and catch up on everything he had missed out on, both academic and athletic. This is another example of finding a learning disability not recognized as such, but once found it was treated and normalized.

It has been found that many adults have wandered through life not even aware of the existence of a classified condition such as dyslexia. Not only have they avoided embarrassing situations because of their inability, but they have avoided anything of a remedial nature. They simply did not know any better. No one had remarked about it, or it was shrugged off or denied by parents. There could be many reasons for a person not being properly cared for, and as time goes on most need seems to cease to exist. This could be one explanation of how the "town dummy" got that way.

There is another category of unawareness—that of gullibility. If the disabled child is cunning enough, and many are, he can con his parents into believing he has no homework. "They didn't give a test today; I was excused from class." All manner of subterfuge is used if it's a case of avoiding an issue, either with parent or teacher. Again, as time goes on, the "lucky" child will reach a point where no one will bother to call him to account at all.

FEAR OF THE NEED TO RETOOL

Some of the adults (from the upper grades of high school and into college) have shown a reticence over being treated for learning disabilities for a valid but unnecessary reason. They have spoken of a fear of having to relearn their way around their difficulties. They have reached a stage of equilibrium in coping and display a strong unwillingness to try anything new that might make them feel unsure of themselves. For them, the unknown can be devastating.

When these patients finally are convinced that nothing but good can come of the treatment, they accept with reservation and then suddenly realize that (in most cases) they "have been reborn and can see and hear their environment properly for the first time."

One case in particular was very exciting, not only for the patient but also for the thirty or so witnesses. A college girl had volunteered quite unwillingly to be the subject of a demonstration for the treatment of dyslexia. She stated a real fear that if it worked, she would have to learn new tricks to get by. In the meantime, she had dropped all courses that involved laboratory work because of her inability to focus a binocular microscope unaided. For her lecture classes, she was depending upon tapes. This would give her the opportunity to memorize by rote so she managed to keep her head above water and passed, but not well.

The demonstrated treatment was accomplished in about twenty minutes. When she was finished, she left the room suddenly, to the surprise of everyone. She ran down the hall, three of her friends after her. Her first stop was to a microscope. Within seconds, her voice rang out, "I did it, I did it! I've focused a single image just like that. I did it!"

The whole class was jubilant over her happiness. Fortunately, her concern over having to restyle her activities was overcome by a stronger desire to be helped, so a happy ending was the result.

On the other side of the coin, however, is the case of a twenty-three-year-old male who has refused all suggestions from friends and family to seek aid. He has stated that he could not face another disappointment in case the care didn't work. He has been through many thousands of dollars and countless procedures only to find no success at all.

BAD-SEED SYNDROME

How many times has one heard the remark, regarding someone not so bright or with emotional problems, "There's bad seed in that family, somewhere," or words to that effect. This may be entirely true because of faulty genetics that follow the tree through several generations. It may be brought about through close intermarrying or certain genetic peculiarities of specific races or peoples.

Most times, however, this is not the case. Although learning disabilities and dyslexia seem to run in families, no demonstrable genetic link has been documented up to the present with the exception of three postmortems that are purported to exhibit a slight distortion in a critical fold in the brain with some displacement and migration of brain cells in one of the interpretation areas. Information on this small sampling is inconclusive but could account for a small percentage of patients who do not completely clear or still have the tendency to reverse.

We find, instead, what seems to be an acquired learning disability which probably came about by disturbing the chemical, neurologic, or structural balance, either prenatally, during the birth process, or traumatically in early life. The distinguishing or differential diagnostic faults present in a dyslexic are not genetic in origin. There are common neurologic or structural faults that, in certain combination, produce a learning disability. Fortunately, all these faults are essentially correctable, and for the most part, when the structure is corrected, the function is corrected.

The thought here of "bad seed" is completely unfair and invalid. If the triad interference had not occurred, the person would have developed as normally as anyone else. To cast the stigma upon someone, in any case, is, of course, not to be done but, when undeserved, is the height of malicious unkindness.

Learning disabilities are not to be ashamed of. They are common problems which should be recognized, admitted to by the parent, and helped as soon as possible. These conditions are treatable and remediable, and, if recognized early enough, the special teaching techniques developed in recent years are of tremendous help.

GUILT TRIP AND DENIAL

Strange as it seems, there are some parents who will avoid facing up to the issue with every fiber of strength in them for an erroneous reason. They are in the belief that they have produced a defective offspring. They have charged their own constitution with the responsibility, and as time goes by, the guilt piles up, higher and higher. The odd part of this is that very often the awareness disappears, while the underlying fact becomes a crutch, thus enabling the parents to bear the disappointment more equably. In order to protect themselves from "attack," they will accumulate a great deal of "feeling sorry for oneself," will cry copious crocodile tears, and eventually will be quite able to deny that anything is amiss.

To reach these parents is next to impossible. Something must happen for the true need to come to light. Often, the one who felt most guilty about the defective child is in great need of care himself or herself. If these parents are denying the problem in the child, imagine how much more in the closet they themselves are! They have had years to learn how to barricade themselves. After all, "What would the neighbors say?"

The Orton Society, formed many years ago for propagation of

information dealing with and for the learning disabled, holds meetings for its members on a regular basis. The authors' attendance at one such meeting resulted in a rather mysterious encounter. An adult female took issue with the speaker. She argued that, "Yes, I do bump into things quite often, yes, I do lose my way trying to follow directions, and, no, I do not know my right from my left hand but surely I'm not dyslexic. I was a straight-A student in college." No one wishes to take issue with her scholastic grades, but one does wonder what her reason for being there was. There were many other things she could have done that evening. Why, one must ask, did she feel compelled to attend a seminar on dyslexia, which she didn't have, according to her own statement? It would be much easier to believe that she was there more as a dual-personality individual. Half of her had come for help, seeking any possible solution to a problem her innermost being knew she had. The other half rebelled, not wanting to let go of what she had accomplished and surely not wanting to admit to others that she was anything other than perfectly normal.

Half of her had won half the battle. She was there. The other half came close to upsetting the applecart by striking out at the one person who might be of help to her. Perhaps some day, in the foreseeable future, she will reach out again for assistance.

There is a situation far worse than denying one's own condition, and that is the refusal to accept the child's problem. There just can't be any feasible excuse for cutting the legs from under another human being who surely deserves every opportunity of care and consideration that is possible. As one mother put it, and she was most sincere, "If I heard that a man standing on the corner dressed in chicken feathers thought he had an answer to my child's disablement, I would break a leg getting to him, and I would thank him profoundly for trying, even if not successfully!"

Another instance of denial came from a schoolteacher. She stated that, of her four classes of thirty children each, she did not have one single learning disabled child! A hundred and twenty children without any problem and this in the face of the documented fact of one out of five of us *with* the problem, small or large.[1-2] She is indeed a lucky and gifted teacher. Incidentally, there was no special education program in her district. Every child was mainstreamed, the theory being that it would tend to raise the level of the slow ones by their exposure to the high achievers. When it was pointed out that this teacher's classes all were divided into fast, medium, and slow groupings, it became clear where the learning disabled were hiding.

12

No Man's Land

Could anything sadder be imagined than the picture of the learning disabled child looking wistfully out the window of his room at the other kids on the block? He has been called "dummy" and "retard." He has suffered the frustration and hurt of not being chosen to play on the sandlot team. He does his classwork poorly and his homework carelessly, and he is forever at odds with his teachers and parents.

At dinner one night, when told to leave the table for slovenly manners, he grabs a gooey dessert, throws it at his brother, who, incidentally, is younger and smarter and much better behaved, glares at his father, turns tear-streaked eyes toward his mother, and stalks out. When he reaches the stairs, he stamps on each one on the way up to his room. His "last word" is the house-shattering slam of his door. Does the reader recognize anyone he or she knows?

Mother looks beseechingly at Father. Father looks disgustedly at Mother. The gauntlet is now thrown. Mother is wondering whether Father is going to whip *her* son. Surely he has the power and the muscles to accomplish it. Father is wondering if Mother is already planning to sneak up to *her* son after he punishes him, to kiss away the hurt and the tears. She certainly has the empathy for it.

If either stopped to consider that the boy upstairs was *their* son, that his heart was breaking, that he had difficulties he didn't understand, another human being might be saved from mediocrity. They might sit down and discuss the problem calmly or perhaps seek advice from someone more knowledgeable than they.

Their son's peers avoid him sometimes because he talks too much, sometimes because he doesn't talk at all. Perhaps he picks fights, perhaps he pits one child against another and then walks away from his devilish handiwork, totally unconcerned.

The three Rs are problems he knows he has, but the social difficulties cause the boy far more immediate grief. Surely he is more affected by the way he is put down, avoided, and shunned by his potential playmates, than by the fact that sometimes a "rat" becomes a "tar" and a *d* becomes a *b*.

Betty Osman, who has written excellent books on the subject of learning disabilities, said it all when she titled one of them, *No One to Play With.*[10]

The child who is lacking in the social graces ends up being ostracized by his peers, which results in nonexposure to any opportunity he might have to learn like the average kids around him have.

One of the horrors of growing up with a disability like this is that of peer pressure, and that is not to say that the child is trying to conform as others do. The fact is that the so-called friends seem to be dedicated to the proposition that anything they can think of to make the disabled more uncomfortable is the thing to do. They will laugh at mistakes, sneer at mishaps, throw all variety of slurs, and, in general, make life a veritable hell for the unfortunate. The more pressure they exert, the worse the disabled child acts, and the worse he acts, the more pressure is thrown at him. Children, dear as they are, can be absolute beasts in the way they treat one who falters. In the tropical fishtank, the one who is in ill health will be destroyed before the day is out. With them that is the law, but with humans there should be more amity exhibited, and one must wonder why this isn't so in more instances than are possible to imagine.

When parents care enough, they can often manage to work out things with their offspring's companions. It is most important that they take and keep control because the child is bound to hurt the one he likes most—his present friend. When that happens, another friend must be found who, it is hoped, will stand by for a reasonable length of time until the cycle repeats itself. If this fact is recognized and dealt with by frank and open discussion with the children involved, there is a good chance the problem will go away.

Following kinesiological correction, the social weaknesses tend to disappear along with the academic ones. The child's feelings are strengthened; his belief in his own worth increases. These facts reflect in improvement in reading comprehension, arithmetic, and general appraisal of his surroundings. Instead of the inverse neurologic, chemical, and structural factors pulling him down, making him lose ground continually, he now has the horse pulling the cart—the neuro-chemico-physico triad is working *for* instead of against him.

One of our eleven-year-olds, Diane by name, had a dangerously explosive situation brewing within her. She knew it but, in her words, seemed powerless to alter it. Any odd look or word out of the way or even an accidental bumping into would result in instant retaliation. Hardly a day went by without Diane being hauled into the office for reprimand because of fighting. It reached the point where, like the "fastest gun," everyone with a chip on his or her shoulder felt obliged to try her out—see if she really was the fastest. Fortunately it was only with fists, but even they can cause a fair degree of injury on occasion.

Several weeks of treatment were necessary to curb the insatiable need to fight, even long after the scholastic skills picked up, but the last and bottom line in this case is that Diane does not look for fights anymore. She has now realized the futility of fighting and is funneling her energies in more useful channels.

Another child, Lisa, had an entirely different situation facing her. She recognized her failings scholastically and outdid herself in developing the most attractive appearance and personality possible. She was a lovely girl, very popular, and rarely had enough time left over from her social whirl to do any important studying, even if she were able. The windup of her case was that she retained the popularity and gathered in the award for most significant scholastic improvement in her senior year at her graduation ceremonies.

This was another example of a child discovering what he or she is best at and concentrating wholeheartedly in that direction. It bears repeating that no two learning disabled are entirely alike. What one doesn't have will shine from another. The financial wizard will not be able to do a book report, but the librarian, who has read avidly all the classics, can't balance her checkbook.

13

Parental Response after the Fact

A short time after the learning disabled patient is discharged as clear, the true measure of the parent becomes known. Some are elated, privately jumping up and down with happiness. They are overjoyed, seeing the child prospering, improving, excelling in all the areas that previously had been such a challenge. These are displays of well-guarded personal pleasure, and if one were to listen carefully, one could hear the sounds of merriment.

There are some who, in addition to feeling strongly, are anxious also to have others share with them and enjoy the tremendous release that kinesiological treatment can give them. They will speak to their friends and tell anyone who is willing to listen what wonderful things happened. One mother in particular had spoken to her church pastor, the child's school nurse, and the school psychologist in the hope that they might know someone else with the same need.

There are still parents who are hostile, disinterested, uncaring, cold to the fact that the child has gone through years of being put down, made fun of, missing the beauty of the printed word. Those not having the disability cannot imagine, in the smallest degree, what the child has to bear. Growing up and developing normally is not that easy, but when a disablement is added, the efforts become almost insurmountable. One patient who no longer needs his parents' help in homework assignments has been accused of letting his work slide. They don't believe he can manage without them.

The foregoing depicts responses ranging from zero to one hundred percent and everything in between. It is hard to imagine anyone who finds it so difficult to be pleased for someone else, especially when that someone is a child, and his or her own child to boot. These people, however, are balanced off by the others who are enthusiastic and make all the attention to detail and the caring so very well worthwhile.

Some parents work very closely with their children, scoring them on degrees of improvement and requiring them to account for the lack of same. Nothing goes so far with a child as earned praise, and it should be given as soon as it is deserved. The reverse also is true.

Unfortunately, there are parents so wrapped up in their own affairs that they haven't the time to give of themselves. If they only knew how desperately their attention was longed for by their children, they just might swing their regard around and do the proper thing.

The authors are fully aware of the probability of engendering displeasure from certain quarters with this statement, but that won't change the facts. In order to draw a truthful picture, one must use the right colors; that is what has been attempted here. The blame is not centered on the fact of *having* a learning disabled child. Rather it is for neglecting full care and consideration after the extent of the problem is realized. Every facet should be explored and every available course taken.

If it is gathered from this that the authors are prejudiced in favor of the disabled one, nothing could be nearer to the truth.

There have been several instances reported by parents of children who are enrolled in special remedial classes that are most disturbing. They have remarked, in certain cases, that if the teacher discovers that a child is being treated by kinesiological correction, the air becomes heavy with hostility. There is nothing the child can do right from that moment on. If he drops a pencil, it seems he is the only one in the class who is not allowed to have that happen. A demerit is earned by having the little one's tie askew. Every moment is dogged by the teacher, who seems to be determined to prove the worthlessness of the procedure. If there is any lapse in the child's deportment or proficiency, the teacher will find it!

The authors have been alerted to the fact that there are two school districts whose jurisdictions are side by side. One is showing a total acceptance of the help available and with gratitude, while the other is reacting entirely in the reverse. Admittedly, school districts enjoy a certain degree of autonomy and so they should, but there is a big question as to whether one would have the privilege of denying help to those who so desperately need it.

There is an example of a family of eight who are selling a large, comfortable home in one township and obtaining another in a different location simply for the purpose of changing school districts. They feel their children are being shortchanged, and they are heading for schools that offer more cooperation. Two of their boys have checked out clear with no more symptoms of being disabled. The school would not recognize the fact and had already signed up the children for continued remedial training at the same level as heretofore. This was done with no further evaluation. No one argues with the fact that the treatment didn't teach the child anything. This is true; the plus derived is that of now being *receptive to being taught.* That fact certainly cannot be a threat to the teacher's security. If anything, it should enforce it. By the time this now-receptive child has completed a school term consisting of the three Rs, he or she will shine with a whole new enlightenment, and, oddly, the teacher is the only one around at the time to receive the kudos.

Why some of the school districts are so solidly entrenched, without the slightest opening available for someone to insert a new idea, is hard to figure. One would think they would welcome any suggestion that would make their job easier. One would also think they would leap at the chance of helping the unfortunates who have such an uphill trek laid out for them for years to come. Can anyone face his or her conscience if *everything* hasn't been investigated, and we don't mean in someone's opinion—we mean *everything.*

Some of the case histories in this volume have been presented to school authorities, only to be shrugged off as not acceptable. It staggers the mind to see this happen!

Of course, for those who are not aware of something of value being available, there can be no blame. It is only after exposure to a tested procedure, fortified with case histories, that one could look askance at the closed mind, and it is the closed mind that will see to it that the students proceed along orthodox lines for the rest of their school experience. They feel secure in the belief that status quo is always the best. To alter this is to "rock the boat," "make waves." These are threatening gestures and not to be entertained by anyone with any sense! Right? No, it is wrong. The threatening gesture is, rather, the wasting of minds that have the inalienable right to the very best available management and to every known procedure. The threatening gesture is that of refusing to potentiate, with *all* available material, every human being equipped to handle it.

14

Look-Alikes

How many times do we hear, "He's the image of his father," "She's the image of her mother"? One of the reasons for the look-alike is the similarity of the bony structure of the face and head. This means the bones themselves are the same shape, same depth, same apposition, one to another. If all the bones are proportionately and equally balanced, and all sutures are properly movable, there is very little chance of genetic inheritance of a structurally caused learning disability. That is not to say the condition couldn't be brought on by neurologic, chemical, or traumatic mishap at a later date.

If the child shows signs of an organizational problem, however, and has a lot of the feature characteristics of the father, there is a strong possibility that the father had pretty much the same disabilities as the son. This supposition is based on the kinesiological research that has been done up to this point.[14] The skull shape and positioning, the ocular muscle tone, and the cloacal reflex readings stand a good chance of being the same. Since cranial faults usually are demonstrated in the learning disabled, it is felt it is proper to interpret a proportion of these people as having a predisposed familial condition.

A good example of similarity is that of a jaw slung to one side, denoting the possibility of a temporal-mandibular joint dysfunction. This could have a marked effect on the physiologic and/or neurologic functioning of the body, a fact well known and dealt with by the dental profession.

For these reasons, it is doubly important that the parent who takes a negative stand, who attempts to hide from the truth, who minimizes the effect his own disabilities might have on his offspring, who violently shouts his denial of responsibility, should pull back, take stock of the real situation, and should pledge his efforts on behalf of doing everything in his power to help his son. The boy is desperately in need of every bit of guidance and empathy the parent possesses.

Those affected parents who simply deny any failings on their part probably are pretty much disabled themselves. The sad part is that, in most cases, if they owned up to the truth, their cooperation would go a long way toward saving their children from years of trying to cope.

The father who continually throws his weight around, shouts commands, and hurls epithets probably is showing his hostility, which could have been brought about by his knowing that his younger brother, an uncle, a next-door neighbor, or even his wife, perhaps, has more to offer. They might have reaped greater rewards, had bigger and better job opportunities come their way, or even are better liked as human beings. This willful and spiteful man should not look upon his duplication in a son and wonder why the poor boy spends part of his school day in the principal's office for picking a fight, and another part in the nurse's office with a fictitious stomachache in order to duck his math class. What the boy is doing is not of his own volition. He is really emulating his father and doesn't even know he is doing it.

Fortunately, there has been a liberalization of attitude concerning the learning disabled, as they are known today. At one time, they were the place for harboring demons. Later, exorcism was entertained. Still later, we were told all these unfortunates were brain damaged and/or retarded. Before the term learning disabled became the vogue, emotionally disturbed was a common appellation. A learning disability somehow becomes a more easily handled situation. The parent might not be quite so irate and might be more willing to accept the problem when it is explained as somewhat less than a stigma.

Dr. Alan Ross has pointed out, in his very fine book on the subject, that learning disabled children are not physically impaired. His description is very well explained.[15] However, our present research[16] has brought to light some minor but nevertheless very important structural abnormalities which, when corrected, have resulted in complete clearance of all disability symptoms. As each case history under the research auspices shows a return to normal, the kinesiological premise gains just that much more fortification and justification.

The most important truth of all is that this type of treatment does not teach the disabled anything. It opens up the normal avenues of reception by removing the structural blockages that are found upon examination. When this is accomplished, the teaching experts, the remedial procedures, the psychological programs can go full steam ahead.

The big difference now is that the students are able to make sense of the conglomeration of learning and before long are found to be reaching out, grabbing at any and all bits of information. They are literally starved for knowledge and find now that they possess the equipment to absorb it. They are able to reap the harvest from their teachers, take it in in great, lustful gulps, and, never being satiated, constantly ask for additional helpings. Being called dull, stupid, dreamer—these days are gone. We are reminded of the child who was asked to write a short note to a friend. This was to test her for spelling, positioning, and comprehensive content. Previous to this, she had not been able to construct a meaningful thought. The note she turned out is reproduced below along with an initial attempt she had made to negotiate writing her name. Note that the dates are nine days apart.

Lauren
June 25th

Baylis
Room 17

Dr.

Lauren

Dear Doctor Wainwright
thank you for helping me
you did a good Job. You're
the best.

Love, Lauren

(Writing test showed a
radical change in nine days.
Ed.)

6/16/83

Dr.

Lauren

Laurel

Laurel

4 y
Lthea ll
n

N n m

7h m Iam

nr a a

(Date at top was inserted. Ed.)

15

Learning Disability vs Hyperactivity vs ?

There is much dispute among researchers, educators, practitioners, and even parents themselves as to which comes first—the learning disability, causing the child to be hyperactive, or the hyperactive child, well out of control and too difficult for the standard classroom teacher to handle, therefore becoming a candidate for special classes. It would be a terrible shame to have a mind wasted only for the reason that deportment was of a poor grade.

Likewise, if a learning disability is so traumatic to the psyche of the youngster that he just can't handle the pressure, there is strong possibility that his nervous reserve won't allow him to perform as his peers and authority figures would wish. This situation can become magnified to the point that because a kid can't spell, he is reprimanded; very often his frustration causes him to take it out on those nearest to him. They, in turn, retaliate. This causes more frustration so that before long, poor spelling might lead to a jail sentence or even worse if the steps fall in the right places. "For the want of a nail, the shoe was lost."

Does this hypothetical situation sound outrageous, preposterous, impossible? Believe it! It is very possible. It has happened over and over and over again. Consider, if you will, the overpopulated penal and corrective institutions with a heavy preponderance of nonreaders and underachievers who had to have come from somewhere.

Many researchers have come this far with their suppositions, among them the thoroughly analytical writer Dr. Alan Ross, who says, ". . . it may be that both hyperactivity and learning disability are caused by some third factor."[17]

Some fault the disability as being responsible for erratic behavior. Others are certain that hyperactive children, by some strange machination, develop a learning disability. Dr. Ross joins the two as a possibility and speculates as to a.third but unknown entity.[18]

Several years ago, when Dr. Goodheart developed and correlated the principles of kinesiology,[19] he laid the groundwork and planted the seed, which has finally flourished and flowered into that third but now known entity.

In most cases, in a matter of a few days, a good deal of the disability and/or hyperactivity has disappeared for good. The frustration and pain of failure have gone; the child is now searching avidly for things to learn about. He acts like the proverbial sponge.

Dr. Ross speaks of the relationship between hyperactivity and learning disability as not at all clear.[20] The present research within the kinesiological field has clarified this relationship so that the followers of the technique can make short work of establishing the God-given miracle of the ability to learn, retain, comprehend, and give back the wealth of information the capable teaching profession is equipped to impart.

It is very important that the people who work with the learning disabled understand one particular fact. No amount of physical, mental, or chemical correction will add a single item of knowledge to one who has a learning disability. Improving the general condition of the individual does just that. It is a self-serving term. Improving the condition improves the condition. We must look for other improvements when these corrections are accomplished. The patient now should show change in receptivity, attention span, deportment, interest, and, above all, ability to comprehend and hold on to the informational bits that are fed to him, be he young or old.

There is only one place these areas of learning can come from— the teacher. The student is now open for the life experience invasion and probably will keep his instructors on a constant move, trying to keep up with him and satisfy his newfound needs.

One fact that is noticed constantly is the rapidity with which the student absorbs new material; it is strikingly fast. What ordinarily would take months to years can very often require only days to weeks to accomplish.

There is a reasonable percentage of students and parents who think that once the corrections are made, they automatically know how to read, write, do math, and so forth. Then if the first attempts are somewhat hesitant, do not flow easily, or the children are not automatically at the top of the class, they give up. They don't try, and they feel that although other areas are now normal or greatly improved, nothing is changed and they don't learn. They can't recognize that they feel differently, see differently, hear and understand differently, and therefore all they need do is apply themselves. If they were to use their new facilities, they would start to feel the thrill of success, the sense of accomplishment and self-worth. Then the learning process starts to be fun and picks up speed.

Because we have brain potential we never use, we have the innate equipment to become Einsteins, Edisons, et al., but few of us ever reach these heights due to various reasons which we won't go into here. The same holds true for the learning disabled who has been treated. Each has his own idea of interest, his own speed of learning, and his own innate abilities. Therefore, not eveyone will learn all there is to learn, but at least now they can learn what they will.

It is important to reemphasize that in order to learn, one must practice reading, writing, and arithmetic. There are many ways open to us to learn, i.e., by example, by stimulation, by accidental injury, but mostly by repetitious application.

Hopefully, we eventually will reach the stage of never again hearing the words spoken by an actor in a movie made in 1981. He was asked, in the script, by his son's teacher why he didn't read and how he had managed to get as far as he had. His answer, with downcast eyes, was, in essence, "You lie and you cheat and you hide yourself in the hills and fake your way through."

A constant question arises in testing and establishing remedies for the learning disabled. One might ask why so many very serious and hardworking researchers use tunnel vision themselves in their presentation. The one considers only visual perception,[24] while another is concerned only with auditory difficulty. Still another will insist that hyperkinesis is the total cause of every learning problem.

Who is going to choose the lethargic type of child and make that the entire issue?

If a child does not perform well in connecting dots to form a picture, what is the choice? Does it perhaps depend on the direction from which the help is sought? Has he a visual, auditory, or behavioral problem? Or is he so jumpy he can't control the pencil? Or perhaps his mind was wandering so he didn't even hear the instructions.

All of these suppositions are irrelevant. Barring eye, ear, or brain pathology, when the cranial and facial bones are manipulated into their proper positions, when the muscles of the eye are balanced, when the cloacal reflex points and the gait mechanisms are corrected, the learning disabled person will behave. He will read and comprehend. He will receive with his five senses, will organize with his intact nervous system, and will express with his now agile communication equipment. Remedial, special, and opportunity classwork will take on an entirely new meaning. Learning will become the thrill, the excitement, the enticement it is meant to be. It no longer will be necessary to be exposed to the jibes of "dummy," "retard," "stupe," and such.

The highly touted, sophisticated testing (with no end in sight) would no longer be necessary, nor would the staggering expense be heaped on society if those unfortunate enough to become learning disabled could be weeded out at an early age and properly normalized in a quick, entirely natural and noninvasive way.

When Drs. Kemper and Galaburda conducted their surgical postmortems and found tissue changes in the left hemisphere of the brains of two certified dyslexics, the immediate thought that comes to mind is that this change could point to the origin of learning disability. They maintain that these changes are traceable as far back as the sixteenth to twenty-fourth week of fetal development.[28] It is not surprising to read of their discovery.

This can be quite true but for reasons not gone into thus far. When there is cranial subluxation, there can be brought about a compression of cranial contents, thus causing reaction among the cellular structures. This reaction can result in alterations of the brain tissue patterns. Thus we could find the abnormalities as stated.[28]

16

Further Findings

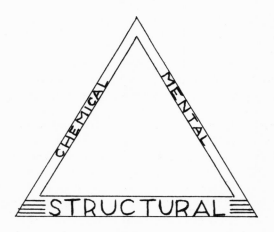

Structural base of the triad

The implications of the structural foundation of the health triad are far reaching and all encompassing. The base of any structure must be level and firmly anchored. The supports must be evenly placed and spaced. They must be strong enough for the job. No amount of mental or chemical contribution will survive very well if the balanced integrity of the foundational structure is found wanting. The importance of the skeletal identity cannot be overemphasized.

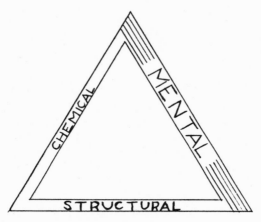

Mental leg of the triad

Just as the structural base of the triad is vitally implicated in the organization of the body and its functions, the mental leg must be considered if we are to treat any condition adequately. Unfortunately, this aspect of health care is either ignored completely or, if taken into account at all, is superficially treated or looked at as a separate entity. Sadly, it is not considered in relation to everything else that is going on or going wrong in the body. This part of the triad was designated "mental" to indicate that it deals with not only the emotional part of the mind but rather its entirety. This includes our attitude, the various mental processes, and our overall approach to life as well.

In the beginning of the treatment for learning disabilities and dyslexia, the authors experienced one hundred percent response on the first twelve cases presented. At that point, unexpected things started to happen. Not taken into account was the tremendous emotional stress placed on the victims. Some patients had partial relief or help but held onto the reversals, or their handwriting didn't improve. One patient's writing got worse. When the emotional factors of the condition were considered, along with the embarrassment, anguish, and frustration they had lived through while growing up, they were able to respond as the others did. A peculiarity was that this seemed to occur more frequently in adult females under treatment as opposed to males or children.

Another important finding that must be emphasized is that emotional factors can reestablish part of the initial problem. A number of children had completely responded and were doing well in school, sports, and social interaction when the condition completely reversed. All or most of the original symptoms returned. On the face of it, it would seem that the treatment was something less than perfect. It had not held and the parents were discouraged. Their reaction was that the period of normalcy was shortlived and the help was only temporary. Upon questioning, it was discovered that in each case the child had suffered severe emotional trauma. It should be stressed that only part of the condition returned, such as the reversals, difficulty in scanning, short memory span, and confusion in comprehension. This, unfortunately, was made doubly distressing because there had been the hiatus from those symptoms for a period of time. Once understood, this can be quickly and easily corrected and the patient normalized again. This is an important factor in many difficult conditions presented to the kinesiologist.

In cases of learning disabilities and dyslexia, emotional trauma produces specific cranial faults which then must be corrected while holding the emotional concept in mind.

The repercussions of this technique are most exciting in the treatment of a multitude of problems, especially the pain conditions that resist the usual approaches of standard medicine, chiropractic, and other healing arts.

In considering the chemical aspects of the triad, we are speaking of the nutritional necessities of healthy living. We must eat correctly in order to be healthy. There is no argument today that you are what you eat. Nutrition has become one of the bywords of good health. Even the most adamantly opposed disciplines of the healing arts finally have come around to recognize this simple truth.

Conditions such as hypoglycemia (low blood sugar) and hypothyroidism (low thyroid output) have long been recognized as chemical imbalances in the body. They can cause fatigue, confusion, loss of concentration, erratic behavior, and loss of comprehension. Some of the same symptoms are found in the learning disabled. In

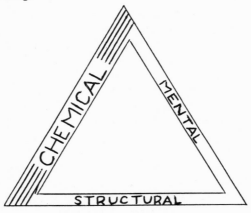

Chemical leg of the triad

learning-disabled and hyperactive persons, it has been found that by supplying a nutritious diet, devoid of the refined sugars and other devitalized substances such as white flour, white rice, and so forth, the child or adult responds dramatically. Particularly important in this concept is a nutritious breakfast. This is not one consisting of a sugared, refined cereal, juice, and white toast or doughnut. Rather let it be one of whole grain cereal, an egg or other protein source, fruit, and whole grain bread. This is good, provided there are no allergies to these particular foods, of course.

We now arrive at the most important part of the chemical area to be considered—allergies. Brain allergy has been recognized for some time, and this is dramatically associated with learning disabilities. Unfortunately, some of these allergies involve what can be considered, for the average person, very good foods, including milk and eggs, whole wheat, corn, and certain fruits and vegetables such as potatoes, eggplant, tomatoes, peaches, and apples.

Chemical allergies, such as those associated with hydrocarbons, also are widespread and have been shown to be related to conditions *similar* to learning disabilities, as well as the actual learning disabilities and dyslexia, specifically. The toxic effects of auto emissions, industrial discharges, cleaning fluids, and solvents used in ballpoint pens and magic markers are some of these.

There has been much discussion about food additives, preservatives, and coloring materials in recent times, and it is accepted by many allergists that these substances are responsible for many behavioral, personality, and disability problems prevalent in our society today.

Dr. Alan Mandell, of Norwalk, Connecticut, has been doing rather dramatic work in this area. Brain allergy must be considered as a major factor in some dyslexic and learning disability problems.

As with emotional trauma, chemical affectation such as allergic reaction creates or recreates certain cranial faults which are treatable or correctable. A case in point is that of Jason, a seven-year-old boy who was seriously hyperactive. This was caused by specific allergies. Sugars and junk foods were eliminated from his diet and the hyperactivity ceased. He responded almost immediately to the structural correction and was doing quite well in school. One day the hyperactive phase returned. With questioning, it was determined he reacted to the pink coloring of bubble gum and a cupcake with pink icing. After the structural and neurologic corrections that were necessary were made, Jason was asked to write his name. It is reproduced below just as he wrote it.

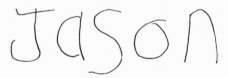

He had a habit of writing his name backward before he was treated.

A tiny piece of the bubble gum was placed under his tongue. He immediately became hyperactive. In attempting to write his name again, after much indecision, he wrote:

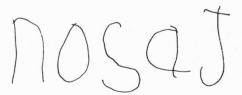

The correction of a tipped sphenoid bone was then made. He immediately quieted and was able to write his name properly:

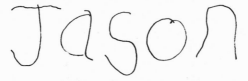

At this point, a small bit of the pink icing was placed under the boy's tongue. He again became hyperactive but slightly less intense. When asked to write his name again, he hesitated and then wrote:

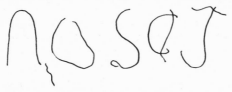

Palpation again located the tipped sphenoid bone. A correction then immediately normalized the neural hangup and the boy wrote:

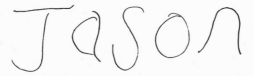

All of the above testing and treatment was in the elapsed time of fifteen minutes. It was interesting to note how rapidly the above changes took place. This dramatically shows the interrelation of chemical, structural, and neurologic action in health and disease.

It has been estimated that up to forty percent of dyslexics are hyperactive and/or chemically reactive. It is obvious, therefore, that diet and allergy analysis are most important in the approach to treatment. The immediate reaction of reversals and confusion resulting from chemical stress has been observed by the authors. Upon palpation examination, specific sphenoidal subluxation was seen to occur at the same time.

The fact that the structural cranial correction could instantly change and neutralize the emotional and/or chemical reaction which recreated the reversals, shows the precise nature of the analysis and treatment.

NOT ALL DYSLEXICS CAN'T READ

An interesting phenomenon has developed in our investigation of certain patients with learning disabilities and, specifically, dyslexia. In the full body examination of patients for the cause of the problem that brought them to our offices, occasionally we have discovered the dyslexic components, i.e., switching, cranial faults, and ocular lock phenomena. When we ask the patients if they have reading problems, they state they read very well and, in fact, enjoy it. They admit to frequent reversal of words and letters, but it doesn't seem to interfere with their ability to comprehend what they read, nor does it create inhibition in wanting to. They accept this situation as normal, although typing and writing are sometimes a problem.

Upon further questioning, as previously stated, we do find they have the directional problems to some degree, the discoordination, and a certain amount of misjudgment in that they tend to bump into things more frequently. They avoid sports that require hitting or catching a ball.

This points to a greater number of actual dyslexics in the population, as these people are often omitted from the statistics. They somehow learned to recognize the code of the words, whether forward or backward. No emotional factors entered in as a child; there were no chemical considerations involved in their problem, and they were able to cope with the world around them.

One eleven-year-old girl was questioned in this area because the dyslexic components were present. She was an honor student, enjoyed reading, and just assumed that everyone saw words, letters, and numbers reversed now and then. When writing, she did not reverse but many times would mix up the sequence of letters. She also professed to be able to read words that were upside down or backward. She joined the gymnastic team in school for the purpose of attempting to overcome a condition of clumsiness. She tended to be absentminded on occasion. This pointed to a possible short-term memory problem.

Normally, these patients suffer from headaches or have vague complaints as opposed to specific problems, indicating neural disorganization.

Another patient presented a peculiar set of circumstances. She too manifested all of the dyslexic components, and when questioned as to having a reading problem or showing a tendency to reverse, she responded with a definite no. She read well, enjoyed it, and experienced no reversals. She was good in spelling and wrote with no effort. She did, however, admit to bumping into things, getting "lost" going around the corner, not knowing right from left most of the time. Only upon fatigue or under nervous stress would she experience a "lazy eye," as she called it, which would then render her incapable of normal reading or writing. She would not be able to scan the printed line properly, would lose comprehension, and in some cases not know what a word was. This type of dyslexia shows up only under certain circumstances but can be found in the structure and, once found, can be corrected. This person's quality of life can be improved by expanding her options so that she can function normally under any conditions.

17

Conclusions

Some researchers have termed forms of learning disabilities as "developmental lags." The authors prefer to think of them as a disorientation between the right and left brain. The defined lag would allude to a slowdown—a child who will "grow into his ability," given sufficient time. If there is disorganization, no amount of time elapsed is going to change anything. The disorganization must be corrected before the child can understand properly what he sees. When this occurs, the letters, numbers, words, and signs will stand still, and he will be able to focus on a single image. Nystagmus will disappear.

Damage and impairment generally are confined to cranial faults, positive cloacal reflex findings, ion discrepancy, and ocular muscle imbalance. None of these is a mental or retardation problem. They are strictly structural.

When all these corrections are made, instruction will be gobbled up.

Everything has a reason. Everything has a cause. Every cause has an effect. Dyslexia and other learning disabilities are conditions just like any other. When taken as a total body or total person problem, as opposed to one that is segmented, they yield to understanding, treatment, and remediation.

Dyslexia and other learning disabilities are multifaceted conditions that show one or many faces in a particular individual. Underneath, however, there is basic discoordination and confusion in the normal reset neural mechanism which allows us to adjust or reorient ourselves to our environment. There seems to be a genetic link in those who don't easily do this, and conditions like dyslexia result and seem to "run" in families. The genetics, so far, do not seem to have any pathology linked to them although one researcher indicates a "kink" in certain brain tissue that may be responsible. In any event, the condition responds almost miraculously to proper treatment. From the beginning, this special procedure provided the desired results. When a problem developed in certain patients, and they did not fully respond, the cause had to be found and then successful correction followed. Emotional factors had to be determined in some. Different factors had to be looked for in others. Food and other allergies had to be considered in certain patients so that, eventually, total correction could be accomplished in each case.

As feedback comes from thousands of patients, more problems will be found besides those already encountered and will need further investigation. Everyone is an individual.

It is best to be reevaluated every so often to make sure all circuits are holding, particularly the corrected cranial faults.

Fatigue, serious illness, overindulgence, and certain injuries can cause some of the switching or centering mechanisms to fail. This could cause a reestablishment of some of the original symptoms. It is important not to be discouraged when or if this happens but to return for treatment. Correction will again provide a state of normalcy.

It is likewise important to think logically about a disability, whether it be learning, physiological, structural, or whatever. If a person is careless about exposure, there is good reason to fear catching a cold. Running afoul of our environment can cause us to catch a learning disability in the same manner. Therefore, we should be checked out periodically for any underlying causes that might be lurking.

The learning disabled will exhibit one or two sphenoidal faults in combination with a positive cloacal reflex and a probable ocular muscle lock. The dyslexic, as a comparison, will show three or four sphenoidal faults, at least one temporal fault, as well as a collection of other reflex failings.

* * *

Most learning disabled have responded in a positive way in one to three treatments and have remained clear on a schedule of bi-monthly reinforcement visits. The full-fledged dyslexics have required five to eight treatments of a more far-reaching nature and have been placed on a biweekly schedule of investigation and correction, if needed.

*   *   *

If the parent or teacher notices any combination of the following signs, there is a fairly certain chance that the child has a learning disability:

1. Constant bumping into people or things.
2. Right- and left-hand confusion.
3. Letter and word reversals in script and/or printing.
4. Marked hesitation in reading and/or talking.
5. Abnormal walking or running. (Cross-switching of arms and legs absent.)
6. Short memory or attention span.
7. Confusion in understanding directional signs.
8. Inability to follow instructions or directions.
9. Poor visual and/or auditory comprehension.
10. Poor mathematical comprehension.

Proper kinesiological investigation and treatment should be sought at early opportunity. The beneficiary will be the child for the remainder of his/her life.

*   *   *

Adults have responded well to the same care but with somewhat more time required. The business of merely living, with the concomitant stresses, places a toll on the person. The number of years of the condition governs, to a degree, the rapidity of response.

*   *   *

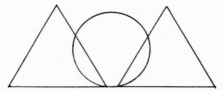

An interesting coordination and organizational test was discovered, and it led to some amazing outcomes. It is reproduced here. The test is to look at the diagram for a few moments and then draw it without looking at it. Next, attempt to draw it while actually looking at it.

Some of the patients trying this have, amazingly, drawn the diagram more faithfully while looking away than while staring at it. This, in itself, most certainly points to the fact that disorganization occurs in direct proportion to the number of actions the body is called upon to perform. In this case, it is a matter of looking and drawing simultaneously, rather than merely drawing alone.

This is not meant to be a trick of any kind. If a person has no degree of learning disability, the diagram test should come out perfectly.

*   *   *

When is a yawn not a yawn?

The average person knows full well that when he yawns, it signifies a sleepiness. If that were the case, why would an animal yawn when he wakes?

The facts are somewhat different. The cranial bones, the cerebrospinal fluid and the venous circulation are directly affected by a yawn. The diaphragm is hooked to the sphenoid and occiput bones by ligaments. Upon yawning, the diaphragm depresses, tugging on the sphenoid and occiput, rocking them both downward.

The temporal-mandibular joint is activated by the yawn as well as the temporal bones.

Many learning disabled tend to yawn much more than the average person. Obviously, it is an attempt on the part of the body to reorganize and revitalize itself. There are many actions that we do instinctively, not necessarily knowing why we do them or even *if* we do them, but the body knows of the need. Fortunately, we have the equipment to bring this about involuntarily, for if we had to rely upon our memory only, there would be many times, no doubt, when we would forget or even defer until more convenient. The body economy would certainly suffer under those circumstances. Nature made sure the many facilities were built into the plan so as to afford an acceptable survival ratio. We even have failsafe backup systems which fill in when needed. It is when the primary system defaults, and the secondary backup gives way as well, that we must call for help.

The various conditions that have been under discussion in this work have not been of a pathologic nature, not that this fact rules out entertaining them as an entity. Oftentimes, a case will be brought in that doesn't match the symptomatic pattern we have been studying. This doesn't necessarily close the door on an effort to help, however. If there is any possibility that findings point in the direction of applied kinesiology technique, no time is wasted. Immediate examination and determination are undertaken and are followed by proper treatment.

A case of cerebral palsy has been improved by making it possible to reduce Depakene medication to one-sixth of what it had been.

A case of medium brain damage was improved by bringing about the child's newfound ability to draw simple pictures and by causing a normalizing rearrangement of the teeth by correcting the placement of the facial and cranial bones and reorganizing the nervous system.

It is now determined that any condition which involves the structural, mental, or chemical aspects of the human, if not pathologic in nature, can be improved by the application of kinesiological procedures.

Postscript

Most, if not all, people would benefit from the potentiation offered by the kinesiological organizational procedures. It has been established that all segments of the body, involving the structural, chemical, and mental constituents, must be fully balanced for the organism to enjoy prevailing good health and optimum integrity.

There are many reasons for this state to become less than perfect. In most instances, the wonderfully integrated body mechanism can handle the environmental onslaught. On many occasions, however, because of any variety of abnormalities and conditions, a fault occurs. This can be effective enough to cause short-circuiting, functional breakdown, or some other aberration.

In some cases, this condition is shortlived and disappears rather rapidly. In others, the stress is too great, and the body is forced to attempt to acclimate itself to the new situation. This is successful part of the time but, unfortunately, not always.

The body, in the latter instances, falls short of its goals and suddenly finds itself in need of help. Nerves are frayed, digestion falters, and postural appearance sags.

Throughout this book, the authors have stressed the importance of neural and neurophysiological organization. This is, after all, the basis of a relief from the learning disabilities and dyslexia. They know that everyone can benefit by at least some of these basic and fundamental, as well as essential, procedures. Almost every patient presents, to a greater or lesser degree, some neural or neurophysiological disorganization. That is why they have what they have, why they suffer as long as they do, and why, barring traumatic complications, they usually end up with a chronic condition.

Few of us eat properly all the time. Many of us are under some sort of emotional, physical, or chemical stress almost every day of our lives. As a good example, very few of us exercise enough or properly, and we tend to abuse our physical body. From time to time, we do not get enough or proper rest; we tend to lift or move too heavy an object (grocery bags, furniture). Many of us have poor posture, both standing and sitting. We may have too soft a mattress. We may wear wrong or badly worn-down shoes, thereby compounding a stress problem with every step taken. If a person wears down his shoes unevenly, he is in need of structural balance and organization.

The average person, for the most part, will not be aware of the disorganization going on in his body, nor will his doctor. He tends to accept an ache or pain, the lack of energy, the occasional confusion, the frequent headache, the digestive problems as normal. He takes a pill and gets along somehow.

In recent years, this problem has come to the surface in a very noticeable way. Athletic endeavors have become extremely popular and have many devotees. Since John F. Kennedy sent out a call for physical fitness (and fortunately the call was answered loudly, we might add), there has been a tremendous upswing in sports for a hobby, sports for personal achievement, and sports for competitive reasons.

Oddly, there is a "good news, bad news" twist to this. The good news is that most of the candidates have prospered, have improved their lot, healthwise, many times over. The bad news is that some have run afoul of Mother Nature's rules. They have, through carelessness or circumstances not of their doing, developed neuro-musculo-skeletal conditions and have had to curb their activities for various lengths of time. Some have their digestion or breathing affected; some have placed too much stress on the various body segments, while still others get tied up in emotional problems. Any one of the three negative conditions can open up a Pandora's box and must be dealt with definitively.

Kinesiology has a complete answer to these problems and should be utilized at the earliest possible opportunity. It never makes sense to overlook or neglect to investigate a situation which is less than normal. Incidentally, when optimum health is enjoyed, there is no awareness of any individual part or function of the body. Each segment goes along smoothly, not calling attention to itself. The time to be concerned is when we become aware of some certain part, be it muscle, organ, nerve, or bone, which is noticeable in some way. What this negative situation is doing is flashing a danger signal and this should not be ignored.

There is another situation that would profit from applied kinesiological investigation, that of a larger group of athletes made up of those who have acclimated themselves to abnormal circumstances and have gone along with their sport, some not even aware that anything is amiss. These people are, by the very nature of the problem, underachievers. Their potential is far greater than their actual performance, and it is hoped that the opportunity of potentiation will somehow find its way to them. Their facility will greatly increase, their scores will be raised, their timing improved.

The athlete, because of the constant monitoring of his performance, is more aware of disorganization. Because they put a greater amount of stress on themselves, the effects of disorganization and reorganization are more dramatic.

An example of this is that of a patient, Ronald by name, who is into competitive running as an all-consuming sport activity. He had been striving to accomplish the six-minute-mile pace for several years but had never been able to do better than 22 minutes in a 3.1 (5k) mile run.

After special kinesiological survey and treatment for the structural imbalances found, he ran the same 3.1 mile course in 19:57. This cut about 2½ minutes off his best previous time. With further treatment, his time was reduced to 19:12 for the 3.1 mile run.

Ron's comment was that he knew something had happened, and he intends to continue the potentiation procedure. He wants to own that six-minute mile. Accomplishing this goal may not sound spectacular to a lot of runners who do better until it is pointed out that Ron is forty years of age.

Injuries disturb the righting or centering reflexes, unbalance the reactive muscle system, and lock the body's various gait positions. This causes certain muscle groups to be constantly facilitated (turned

on) and certain other ones to be constantly defacilitated (turned off).
A marked example of this was of a baseball pitcher diagnosed as
having a possible rotator cuff tear of his right shoulder. Any attempt
to pitch created much pain and very little control. A kinesiological
examination found his trouble to be a combined gait abnormality
and ocular lock.

There are many causes that bring about an underachiever, be he
athlete or just sedentary homebody. There are those who have had
an automobile accident, those who have fallen off a ladder, those
who have sat down violently while skating. In all such cases, structure
has been altered, muscles have been bruised, nerves have been irritated if not outright damaged. At this point, a long and complicated
adaptative process begins.

As time goes on, the bruises disappear, the physiology does its
appointed job of self-anesthesia, the reactive muscles set up surrogate
stress levels to make up for the deficits. The patient is now satisfied
that the results of the injury are cleared up. Nothing could be further
from the truth. The cloacal reflex mechanism has imprinted a pattern
of insult on the nerve system that will remain until reversed. In no
way will the organism be back to normal until correction is made.

Erratic and unexplained symptoms, such as chronic headaches,
eye strain, nervousness, and any number of other annoyances, will
prevail but have no apparent (to the patient) connection with the
original injury.

When the abnormalities are corrected and the functions are
stabilized, the patients will be shocked to discover how far they have
gone backward since being injured. They also will be amazed to find
how much they have been missing in "feeling good." They have
had no awareness of some symptoms substituting for others. The
surrogate process is slow and somewhat invisible. It creeps along un-
noticed, chipping away at a person's stability. Adaptation of one
part, function, or muscle group to fulfill the need of another will
take place insidiously, leaving the organism shortchanged. Sooner
or later, the lack of our total equipment will be noticed and, eventually, can result in deficit health. At that point, symptoms will
emerge (not obviously related to the original problem). It is here that
the patient will seek help and will be mystified to find that the blow

suffered months ago had contributed to today's complaint.

In conclusion, let it be understood that all systems must be in a state of equilibrium if the organism is to operate at peak performance, and this is true whether we consider birds, fish, animals, plants, or people. Breeding and feeding procedures are very carefully controlled if for no other reason than the effect on the economy in animal husbandry and agriculture. For some reason that eludes us, we are not so careful of ourselves, even when it is so apparent that good health, top performance, and a longer, more productive, more comfortable life would be our legacy.

Applied kinesiology, the latest breakthrough in good health and well-being, has been embraced by several of the health delivery professions but was originally discovered and researched by chiropractors. In order to improve the state the body is in and the way it functions, all aspects of the organism must be in balance. Kinesiology is the procedure by which this is accomplished.

Epilogue

There are still many areas which deserve to be thoroughly investigated by those embracing the specialty. It is hoped that the remaining factors, unknown at this point in time, will be out in the open before very long.

Diligently applied research of a serious nature cries out to be performed. It is hoped that the legacy of accomplishment will fall into the hands of those best equipped, by virtue of curiosity and courage, to bring it about. Great precedent has been posted by all those who have set the pace and traveled the road of sincere investigation. They are to be commended.

The child or adult with the disability will be the beneficiary. Every foot gained in the direction of potentiation will be another milestone toward the goal of perfection.

Dr. R. B. Wainwright

Appendix

There are a few tests that might be tried if the reader knows or suspects he or his child is learning disabled. One is to try the cross-crawl exercise. Lie on your back, raise right leg and left arm simultaneously, then the left leg and right arm. Alternate this for about five minutes. Now attempt reading. It is generally found that there is better clarity and comprehension. This is a small part of the neural organization necessary to correct most of the disabilities.

Another test is to touch the temple area on each side. One, usually the right, may be very tender. You may discover a ridge on the tender side and a depression somewhat lower on the nontender side. This would be an indication of one of the sphenoid faults found in dyslexia. You can thereby start to understand part of the cranial fault mechanism and part of the procedure necessary to make corrections.

Another way to check the sphenoid tilt is to press the tips of the thumbs up against the protrusions located just behind the upper wisdom teeth. If the sphenoid is low on one side (usually the left), the protrusion will appear to be low on the same side as well. These are known as the hamular processes of the lower tip of the sphenoid bone.

Still another test is that of putting pressure on the two K27 (acupuncture meridian) spots, shown in chapter 7, "Examination Factors." If they are tender, rub them lightly until the tenderness leaves, usually two to three minutes. Again you will find reading easier and more readily comprehended.

These simple tests are part of the neural organization or cranial indicators spoken of earlier. If you or your child has the problem, you will find these three as described.

There is, finally, a treatment for dyslexia and learning disabilities. It works most of the time. It only takes a few days or weeks, depending upon the particular patient. It is safe, natural, nonintrusive and very precise.

The ratio of success over the past two years with the patients who have completed the treatment protocol has been too great to ignore. Hence this book.

Bibliography

CF   Fredericks, Carlton, Ph.D., *Low Blood Sugar and You*. Constellation International, 1969. Well-constructed guide to the use of carbohydrates in the average diet.

SP   *Spears Hospital News*. Denver, Colorado, 1952. An informative health news bulletin.

CR   *Congressional Record*, circa 1950. A verbally reported list of findings, read before the U. S. Congress.

1. Goodheart, George, D.C., *Applied Kinesiology*. Privately published. 13th edition, 1979. A technical textbook.

2. Orton Society, Towson, Maryland. Founded in 1949. Listed in organizational directory in public libraries.

3. Clarke, Louise, *Cant Read, Cant Write and Cant takl Too Good Either*. Extremely interesting account of Mrs. Clarke's problems with her dyslexic son.

4. Clifford, Gary, *People* magazine, 1983. Short article as told by Ann Bradford Mathias.

5. Goodheart, George, D.C., *Applied Kinesiology*. Privately published. 10th edition, 1974. A technical textbook.

6. Delacato, Carl H., M.D., *Diagnosis and Treatment of Speech and Reading Problems*. Chas. C. Thomas, Springfield, 1963. A technical textbook.

7. Walther, David S., D.C., *Applied Kinesiology*, vol. I, 1981. A technical textbook.

8. Diamond, John, M.D., *Behavioral Kinesiology*. Harper and Row, 1979. Combined technical and for the lay reader.

9. Goodheart, 1979.

10. Osman, Betty B., *No One to Play With*. Random House, 1982. Well written book for the lay reader.

11. Walther, 1981.

12.   Ibid.
13.   U. S. Dept. of Health and Human Services, *Cesarean Childbirth.* Statistical Reports, 1981.
14.   Walther, 1981.
15.   Ross, Alan O., Ph.D., *Learning Disability.* McGraw-Hill, 1977. For the lay reader.
16.   Walther, 1981.
17.   Ross, 1977.
18.   Ibid.
19.   Goodheart, 1979.
20.   Ross, 1977.
21.   Ibid.
22.   Walther, 1981.
23.   Ibid.
24.   Ferreri, Carl A., D.C., Ph.C., "Dyslexia and Learning Disabilities Cured," *Digest of Chiropractic Economics*, 1983. Article for both the professional and lay reader.
25.   Beasley, Joseph D., M.D., *Impact of Nutrition on the Health of Americans.* Medicine Nutrition Project, Bard College Center. Combined for the lay reader and the professional interested in nutrition.
26.   Ibid.
27.   Frostig, Marianne, Marianne Frostig Center of Educational Therapy. For the lay reader.
28.   Kemper and Galaburda. A surgical dissection team at Boston's Beth Israel Hospital, 1979. Statistical report of findings.
29.   Cohen, B. A., "Role of Eye and Neck Proprioception Mechanisms in Body Orientation Motor Coordination," *Journal of Neurophysiology*, vol. 24, January, 1966.
30.   Magoun, H. J., D.O., *Osteopathy in the Cranial Field*, vol. III. A technical textbook.
31.   Twitchell, Thomas, "Sensory Factors in Purposive Movements," *Journal of Neurophysiology*, vol. XVII, May, 1974.
32.   Turbo, Richard, *Success* magazine, March, 1982. Magazine article for the lay reader.